Cardiac Pacemakers and Implantable Defibrillators:
A Workbook in 3 Volumes

Edited by

David L. Hayes, MD

Paul J. Wang, MD

Volume 1

Cardiac Pacing: A Case Approach

David L. Hayes, MD

Paul J. Wang, MD

Marleen E. Irwin, RCRT

A. John Camm, MD

FUTURA

**Futura Publishing
Company, Inc.**
Armonk, New York

© 1998 by Futura, an imprint of Blackwell Publishing

Blackwell Publishing, Inc./Futura Division, 3 West Main Street, Elmsford, New York 10523, USA
Blackwell Publishing, Inc., 350 Main Street, Malden, Massachusetts 02148-5018, USA
Blackwell Publishing Ltd, 9600 Garsington Road, Oxford OX4 2DQ
Blackwell Science Asia Pty Ltd, 550 Swanston Street, Carlton South, Victoria 3053, Australia
Blackwell Verlag GmbH, Kurfürstendamm 57, 10707 Berlin, Germany

03 04 8 7 6

ISBN: 0-87993-695-9

Acquisitions: Jacques Strauss
Printed and bound by: IBT, Inc., Troy, NY

For further information on Blackwell Publishing, visit our website:
www.futuraco.com

Introduction

This workbook is directed towards physicians, nurses, technicians, technologists, and industry engineers and representatives. It provides a diverse series of problems in cardiac pacing on a broad range of topics. It is based on the principle that learning by doing is the best instruction. The cases have been divided by their level of difficulty: easy, moderate, complex. For each case, a question is given with a tracing or radiograph and is followed by the answer.

EASY

CASE 1

Question:

You are presented with the following tracing from a patient in the pacemaker clinic for a routine visit. The patient is not pacemaker dependent and is asymptomatic. The information you are given is as follows:

Mode: VVI
Lower Rate: 70 bpm

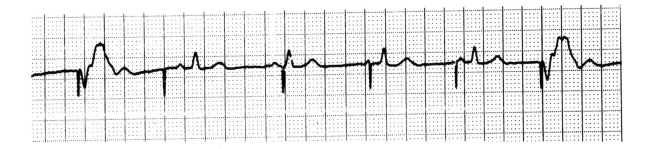

1. List all of the events noted on the tracing.
2. Is pacemaker function normal?
3. Should any programming changes be made?

Sinus rhythm
ventricular capture
ventricular non-capture
functional
ventricular fusion beat

Answer:

1. The following events occur on the tracing:
    Ventricular capture (**1**)
    Ventricular failure to capture (**2**)
    Appropriate ventricular sensing (**3**)

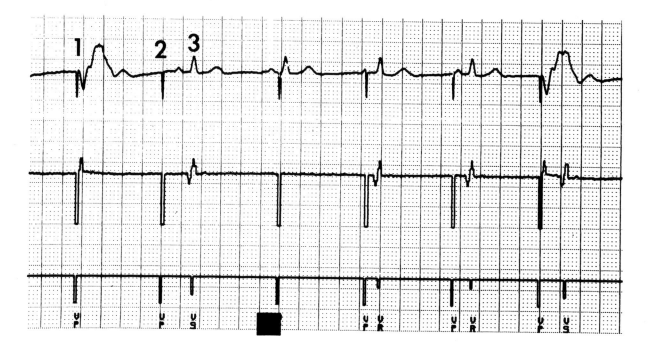

2. Pacemaker function is abnormal with intermittent ventricular failure to capture.

3. Acutely, ventricular voltage amplitude and/or pulse width could be increased in an effort to achieve consistent capture. Ventricular pacing thresholds should be determined in the course of the programming. Differential diagnosis would include chronic rise in pacing thresholds either due to dislodgment, drugs causing a rise in threshold, exit block or loss of lead integrity, i.e. insulation failure or conductor coil "make or break" fracture. Other information that would be helpful would include lead impedance and a chest x-ray.

CASE 2

Question:

You are presented with the following tracing from a patient in the pacemaker clinic for an unscheduled visit. The patient is pacemaker dependent and complains of recent onset of exercise intolerance and fatigue. The information you are given is as follows:

Mode: DDD
Lower Rate: 48 bpm   *1250 ms*
Upper Rate: 120 bpm   *500 ms*
AV Interval: 200 ms

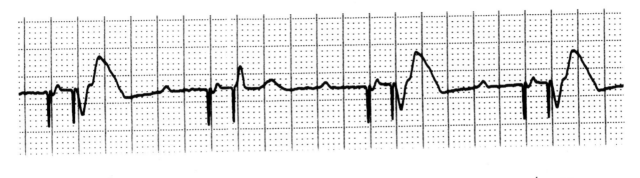

1. List all of the events noted on the tracing.
2. Is pacemaker function normal?
3. Should any programming changes be made?

Atrial NON-sensed beats
Atrial pacing
Ventricular c-pm

Answer:

1. The following events occur on the tracing:
    Atrial capture (**1**)
    Ventricular capture (**2**)
    Atrial undersensing (**3**)

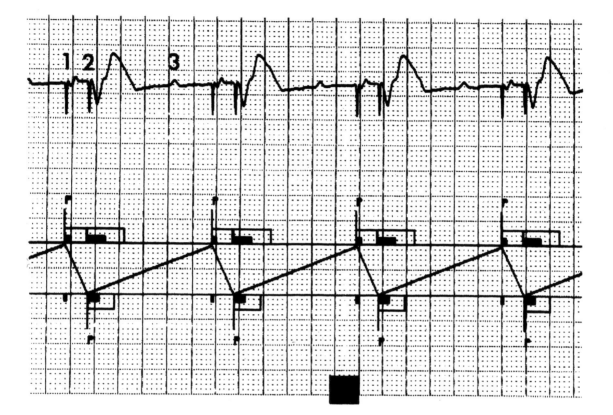

2. Pacemaker function is abnormal with intermittent atrial undersensing.

3. Atrial sensing threshold should be determined. If the atrial sensitivity can be programmed to a more sensitive value it is possible that the abnormality can be corrected. One would also have to consider other clinical information. For example, if this is a relatively recent implant, atrial lead position should be evaluated by chest x-ray. Atrial lead impedance should be checked as a clue to whether there may be a breach in lead integrity.

CASE 3

Question:

The ECG and telemetry data were recorded in a patient implanted with a DDD pacing system 48 hours prior to the recording shown. The atrial output is programmed to 6.0volts at 0.6ms.

What is the most appropriate next step in management?

Battery/Lead Values:

Collected: 3/13/96 14:25

Battery Status: OK
Estimated Time to
  Replacement(Average) 107 months(Past History)
Battery Voltage   2.79 V
Battery Current   13.1 uA
Battery Impedance   100 Ohms

Thera D 7964i/651/661   3/13/96 14:31
CHART SPEED 25.0 mm/s

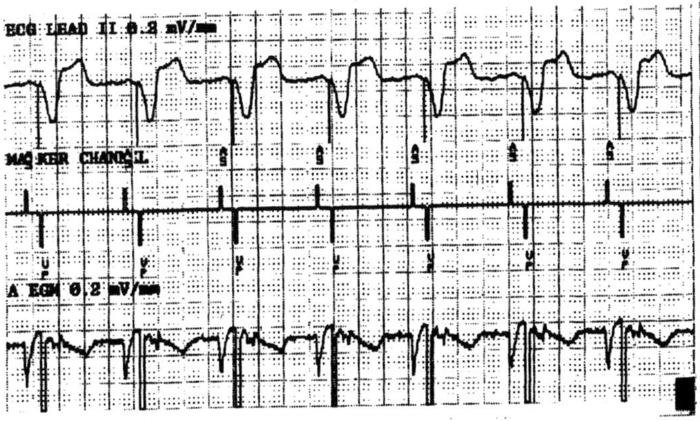

Lead Status:	Atrial	Ventricular
Pulse Duration	0.40	0.40 ms
Pulse Amplitude	4.19	4.07 V
Output Energy	0.0	8.8 uJ
Lead Current	0.0	5.8 mA
Lead Impedance	> 9999	666 Ohms
Pacing Configuration	Bipolar	Bipolar

ECG LEAD II 0.2 mV/mm

MARKER CHANNEL

A EGM 0.2 mV/mm

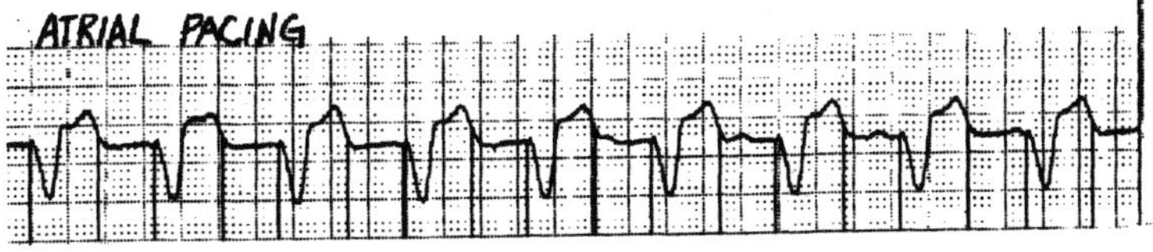

ATRIAL PACING

Answer:

Even with a very high atrial output, loss of atrial capture is evident. With the atrial impedance recorded at > 9999 ohms, the most likely cause of this presentation is that the atrial set screw has not been properly engaged.

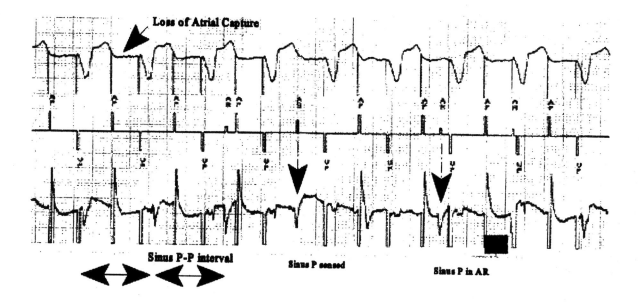

The timing diagram shows that the intrinsic sinus P waves are occurring irrespective of the atrial output. The atrial output is not capturing the atria, thus the intrinsic atrial rhythm prevails.

Final interpretation: Loss of atrial capture; extremely high atrial lead impedance recording due to a loose / improperly engaged atrial lead set screw.

CASE 4

Question:

A 73-year-old female presents to the emergency room with chest pain. There are pacing artifacts on the ECG and you are asked to review the tracing. Chest x-ray is not yet available, but the patient has her identification card. From this, you are able to discern that the patient has a single-chamber pacemaker and the lead-model number given is one of an active fixation atrial "J" lead. The patient tells you that she has a history of paroxysmal atrial fibrillation and that her regular doctor told her that they were going to pace her heart faster than usual in an effort to prevent the irregular rhythm. The rhythm strip obtained in the ER is shown here:

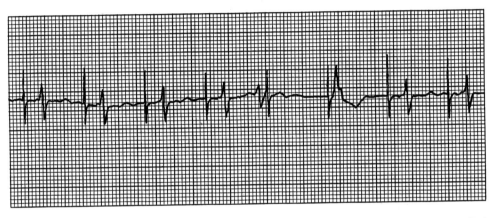

CM712311-01.ai

1. Is this normal function for what is presumed to be an AAI pacemaker?
2. Could a ventricular event appropriately reset the timing cycle of an AAI pacemaker?
3. Is there merit to the way in which the pacemaker is programmed?

atrial capture
AV Conduction
PVC

680ms Pacing artifact

Answer:

1. The ECG demonstrates normal AAI function at a rate of approximately 90 bpm. The 4th and 5th pacing artifacts (**arrows**) occur immediately after and preceding QRS complexes. An AAI pacemaker does not sense or respond to ventricular events and this is, therefore, normal function. It is impossible from this tracing to say if these artifacts result in atrial depolarization. This could be proven with an atrial electrogram.

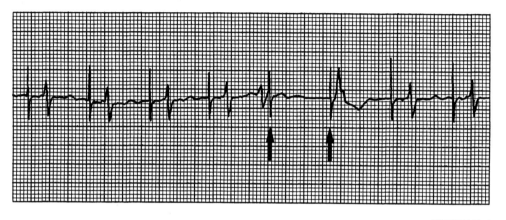

CM712311-01.ai

2. The following simulated ECG tracing demonstrates an AAI pacemaker at a programmed rate of 50 bpm. A PVC occurs with retrograde VA conduction. The retrograde P wave is sensed (**arrow**) and appropriately resets the timing cycle of the pacemaker.

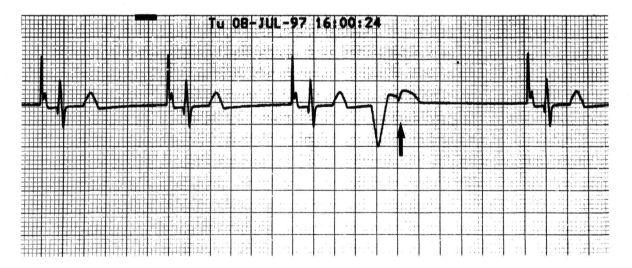

3. There are some clinicians who believe that pacing the atrium at a faster rate, i.e. 80 to 100 bpm, may prevent recurrent episodes of paroxysmal atrial fibrillation. This information is largely anecdotal although trials currently underway may help demonstrate the true value of this method.

CASE 5

Question:

Programmed Settings

DDDR
Lower rate   1091 ms (55bpm)
Upper rate   571 ms (105 bpm)
A-V delay   220 ms
PVARP   340 ms

How do you explain the change in the rhythm?

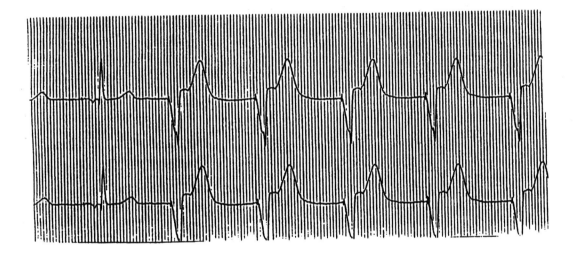

Answer:

There is evidence of ventricular pacing at the lower rate of 1091 ms (55bpm). However, there is no evidence of atrial pacing. Therefore, it is most likely that the mode is now VVI or VOO. This may have occurred through mode switching. For some pacemakers, atrial noise reversion also results in VOO pacing. Following each ventricular paced event, there is probably a retrogradely conducted P wave.

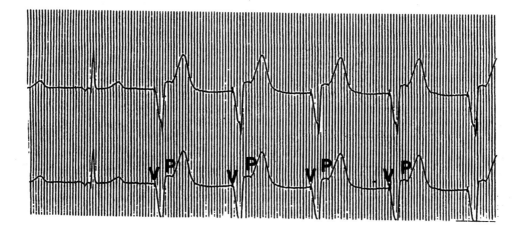

CASE 6

Question:

An elderly male received a VVI pacemaker at your institution 5 years ago. Subsequent follow-up has been performed by his local physician. The patient is sent to you for urgent reevaluation after the following ECG tracing was obtained:

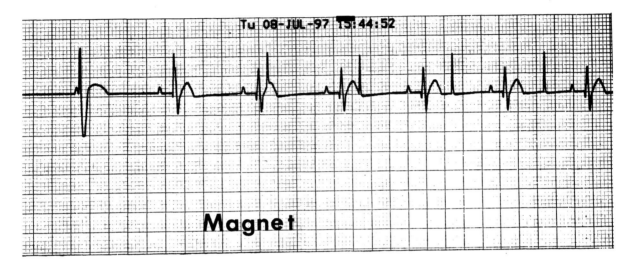

The pacemaker is programmed to a rate of 60 bpm. The patient states that he is asymptomatic.
1. How would you interpret the ECG tracing?
2. What steps should be taken at this time?

Answer:

1. The ECG probably reflects normal VVI function. The ECG is clearly marked as a magnet tracing. The patient is presumably sent with a working diagnosis of intermittent failure to capture. The pacing artifacts that definitely fail to capture (**arrows**) occur when the ventricle is refractory because of the preceding intrinsic QRS complex. This is functional failure to capture, i.e. capture does not occur as a function of normal physiology, the myocardium is appropriately refractory. The artifact marked by the asterisk is probably also functional failure to capture. This artifact occurs at approximately 400 ms after the intrinsic QRS. The duration of the intrinsic refractory period will vary from patient to patient and in some patients the ventricle would be vulnerable to stimulation at 400 ms.

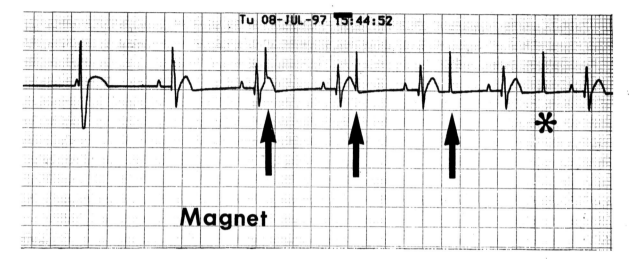

2. Although this is probably normal, the failure to capture the last artifact (**asterisk**) would warrant a closer evaluation to be absolutely certain that capture is normal.

CASE 7

Question:

You are called to assess pacing function in a 72-year-old male with severe depression hospitalized in the psychiatric unit. He has a bipolar DDDR pacemaker programmed to DDIR mode in a bipolar pacing and sensing configuration. This ECG was obtained following electroshock therapy:

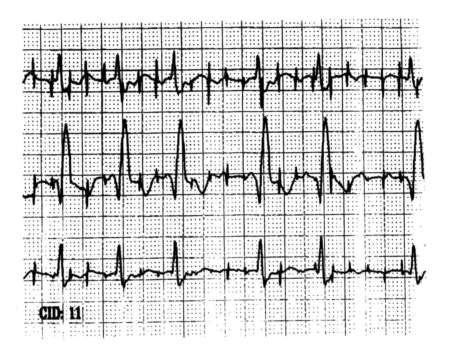

1. Is the pacemaker functioning normally?
2. What can be done to confirm your diagnosis?

Answer:

1. The pacemaker is functioning normally and ECT had no bearing on ECG findings. Artifact created by 60 - cycle interference accounts for the ECG appearance.

2. This interpretation can be confirmed by the use of pacemaker derived ECG interpretation channel (Marker Channel™). The Marker Channel™ for this patient is shown here:

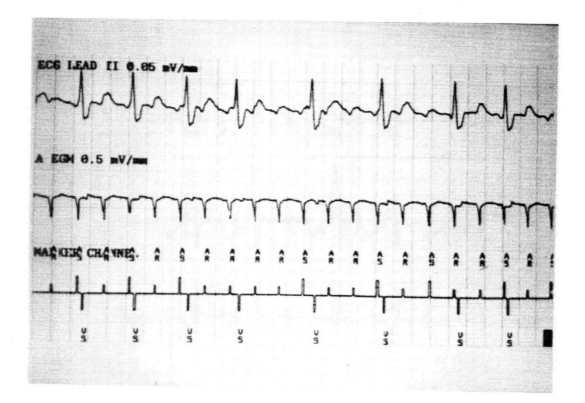

The underlying paced rhythm can be seen without any recognition of the artifact that is so prominent on the ECG.

CASE 8

Question:

Programmed Settings:

DDD

LRL	1000 ms (60 bpm)
URL	480 ms (125 bpm)
AV Interval	200 ms
PVARP	280 ms

What is the underlying rhythm? What determines the ventricular pacing rate?

Answers:

There are P waves (p's) which are in a 2:1 ratio to the ventricular paced events. The atrial rate at which the P waves result in a 2:1 AV response rate calculated by adding the PVARP with the A-V interval. In this case, the 2:1 rate is 480 ms.

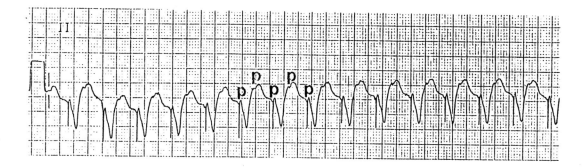

CASE 9

An elderly woman is referred to the pacemaker clinic having never been seen before at your institution. She has no pacemaker identification card and recalls little information regarding her pacing system. A chest x-ray is obtained and is shown below:

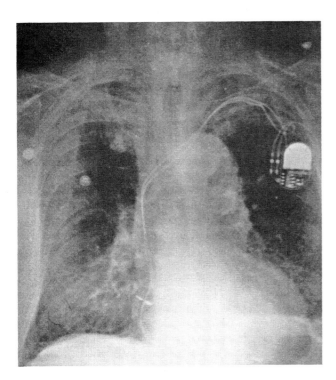 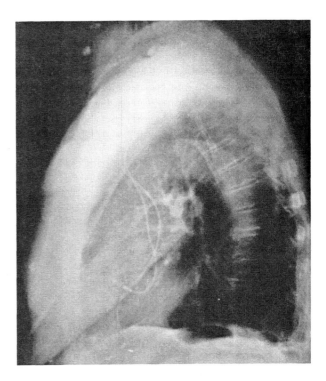

1. Describe the pacing system by trying to detect as many details as possible from the chest x-ray.
2. Can you identify the specific pacemaker manufacturer?
3. How would you proceed in an effort to obtain more information about the pacing system in place?

Answer:

1. The chest x-ray demonstrates a dual-chamber bipolar pacemaker with two bipolar leads. The pacemaker is in a left pre-pectoral position and the course of the leads suggests probable subclavian approach. The atrial lead is positioned anteriorly with an adequately shaped "J." The ventricular lead is positioned in the right ventricular apex.

2. A close-up of the radiographic image of the pacemaker is provided. At one time the radiographic shape of the pacemaker was relatively unique to the manufacturer. This simple observation often allowed identification of the pacemaker manufacturer. As pulse generator sizes have decreased, the "can" design is no longer manufacturer unique.

Most pacemakers do have a radiographic identifier that allows identification of the manufacturer and sometimes the specific model. In this pacemaker, the company logo (Medtronic, Inc., Minneapolis, MN) is seen on top, with the designation "PGJ" under the logo. By calling the company's technical service number (all companies have a toll-free '800' number and most will answer 24 hours/day) the radiographic code can be identified. In this example, PGJ indicates a specific DDDR pacemaker that the technical service identified by name and model number.

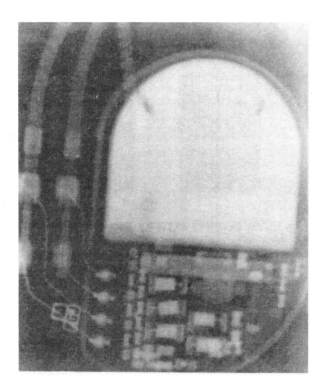

3. Once the pacemaker manufacturer has been identified several approaches can be used. If the manufacturer's programmer is capable of model identification, simple interrogation may provide all of the information needed. All pacemaker manufacturers have a registration department that should be able to provide some information with only the patient's name. Although they may not be able to release some of the information, they should be able to identify pacemaker model, date of implant and possibly lead types. Obviously the implanting physician can be contacted directly if the patient is capable of supplying this information.

CASE 10

Question:

You are presented with the following tracing from a patient in the pacemaker clinic for a routine visit. The patient is asymptomatic. The information you are given is as follows:

Mode: DDD
Lower Rate: 60 bpm   1000m
Upper rate: 110 bpm   545
PVARP: 160 ms

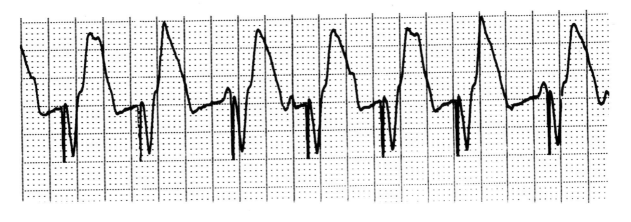

1. List all of the events noted on the tracing.
2. Is pacemaker function normal?
3. Should any programming changes be made?

Sinus rhythm
Ventricular capture
Not ~~atrial track~~

Answer:

1. The following events occur on the tracing:

Appropriate atrial sensing (**1**)
Ventricular capture (**2**)
Pseudo-Wenckebach upper rate behavior

2. Pacemaker function is normal.

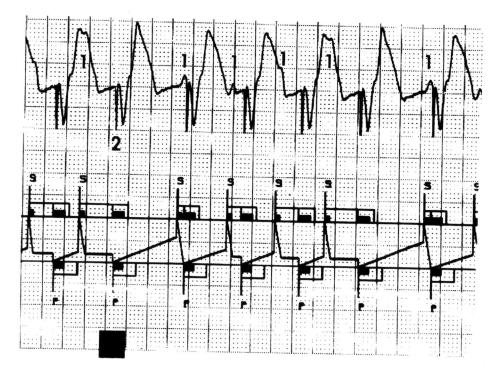

3. This is appropriate upper rate behavior as long as the patient experiences no symptoms when the upper rate limit is achieved; therefore, no programming changes should be required.

MODERATE

CASE 1

Question:

A 66-year-old male with sinus node dysfunction and Parkinson's disease receives a DDDR pacemaker. Six months later he is referred to you for evaluation of paroxysmal atrial fibrillation, which has been difficult to control. When reviewing the pacing history the patient states that he has not had any further syncope but has episodes where he feels "odd" and "just not right" that he never experienced prior to pacemaker placement. Further questioning reveals that this odd sensation occurs most commonly when he bends over to tie his shoes. Programmed parameters are as follows:

DDD
Lower rate: 50 bpm *1200*
Upper rate: 120 bpm *500*
Voltage: 3.5 volts in both chambers
PW: 0.45 ms in both chambers
Pacing configuration: Unipolar
Sensing configuration: Unipolar
Sensitivity: A = 0.8 mV and V = 3.5 mV
PVARP = 200
CVTL = 85

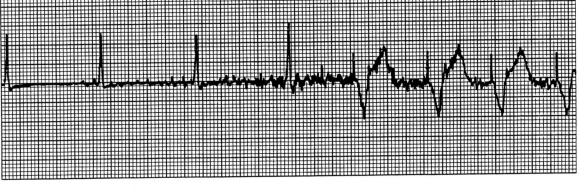

CM721311L-58.AI

1. What clinical approach would you take to evaluate his perceived pacing related symptoms?
2. What is your diagnosis?
3. How would you correct the problem?

Answer:

1. Since the patient can describe a specific maneuver the causes his symptoms it would be reasonable to reenact the maneuver while electrocardiographically monitoring the patient. This was done and the ECG tracing is shown below.

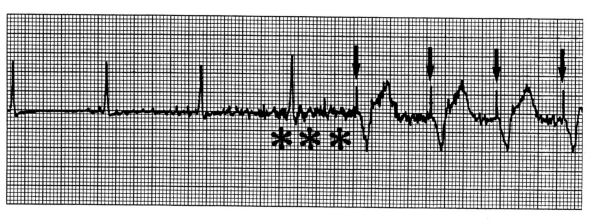

CM721311L-58.AI

2. The ECG tracing reveals significant baseline irregularity during the patient maneuver which represents myopotential induced artifact (**asterisks**). Following the myopotential interference there is ventricular pacing at a rate faster than the intrinsic rhythm at the beginning of the tracing (**arrows**). The ventricular sensing circuit is tracking the myopotential interference that is sensed on the atrial lead. Because the atrial sensing circuit is sensing myopotentials, and not true atrial depolarization, the patient is effectively pacing only the ventricle, i.e. the patient suffers loss of AV synchrony. Symptomatic ventricular pacing in this patient is compatible with pacemaker syndrome. Even though he has a DDDR pacemaker in place this is still pacemaker syndrome and the treatment would be to avoid the mechanism by which AV synchrony is lost.

3. Note on the programmed parameters that this is in a unipolar pacing and sensing configuration. Unfortunately, this was a unipolar pacing system, i.e. no option existed to change sensing polarity. Also note that the atrial sensitivity is very sensitively programmed at 0.8 mV. Sensing thresholds revealed that sensing of intrinsic P waves could be consistently maintained at 3 mV. The pacemaker was reprogrammed to a less sensitive atrial value of 2.0 mV and the original maneuver repeated. Although there was still evidence of myopotential artifact on the ECG, the pacemaker no longer tracked the muscle noise, therefore, the patient continued in NSR.

CASE 2

Question:

Pacemaker Settings:
DDD
Lower Rate: 60 bpm   *1000*
Upper Rate: 120 bpm *500*
AV interval   150 ms
PVARP   300 ms

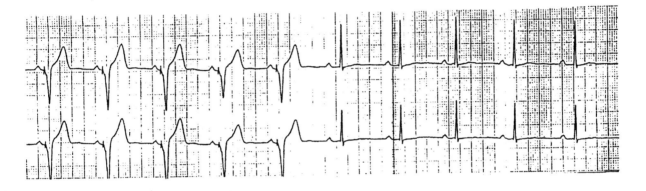

Why are the P waves not followed by paced QRS complexes in the right part of the panel? What are the various explanations? If this observation was due to electromagnetic interference, what would be the most likely explanation?

Answer:

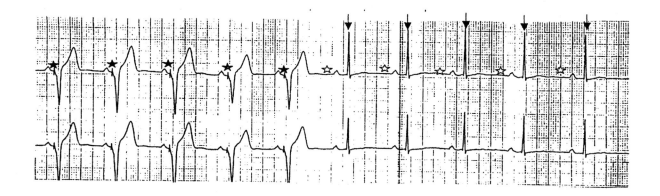

   In the left part of the panel, in the DDD mode, the P waves are followed by paced QRS complexes (indicated by the black closed stars) at the programmed AV interval. In the right part of the panel, the P waves are not followed by paced QRS complexes. Instead, an intrinsic R wave is present (arrows).

   There are several explanations for P waves that are not followed by paced QRS complexes. In some cases undersensing of the P waves may occur because of small P wave amplitude. The QRS must occur within the atrial escape interval, lower rate limit - AV interval, or 1000ms – 150ms = 850ms. Another explanation is oversensing in the ventricle within the AV interval. This would have to occur repetitively always within this interval. Another explanation would be oversensing of the ventricle (open stars) prior to the P wave so that the P wave fell into the PVARP. If electromagnetic interference was the cause either explanation of ventricular oversensing might be possible but atrial undersensing would not be a result from electromagnetic interference.

LRI 631 ms

CASE 3

Question:

A 6-year-old male with complex congenital heart disease develops post-operative symptomatic sinus node dysfunction. AV node function is normal at the time of implant. An AAI pacemaker is implanted and programmed to a rate of 95 bpm. The mother was instructed on how to check her son's pulse and that she should contact the pacemaker clinic if the pulse was less than 95 bpm. She calls to report that her son's pulse has intermittently been less than 95 bpm but that his behavior has been normal and he has no specific complaints. An ECG tracing is obtained:

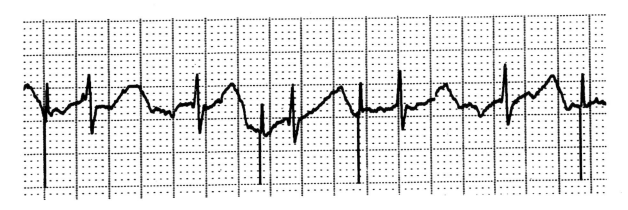

1. Is the ECG tracing normal?
2. What programming changes would you make?

Atrial capture
Long AVI
Ventricular E beats

Answer:

1. The transtelephonic tracing is abnormal. Programmed to a rate of 95 bpm, there should not be an AA cycle length slower than 631 ms. In the tracing shown, the intrinsic ventricular cycle length is slightly longer than expected at approximately 680 ms. The pacing interval can be determined by the AP-to-AP interval near the middle of the tracing. The intervening QRS event is sensed on the atrial channel but falls within the refractory period and is designated "AR" by the Marker Channel™. The same cycle can be measured at the end of the tracing from the last "AS" event to the final "AP" event.

There are two abnormalities noted on this tracing. There is consistent far-field sensing of the QRS. When the QRS is sensed on the atrial channel outside the refractory period, AS, the timing cycle is reset. The cycle is not reset if it occurs in the refractory period, AR. The other abnormality is one of variable AV conduction. After the intrinsic atrial events that occur, conduction to the ventricle appears normal with a PR interval of approximately 180 ms. Conversely, the AR interval (atrial pacing to intrinsic QRS complex), is significantly longer, approximately 240 ms. Given the interatrial conduction delay that occurs after right atrial pacing, the AR and PR intervals may not be effectively different, but the electrocardiographic appearance is striking.

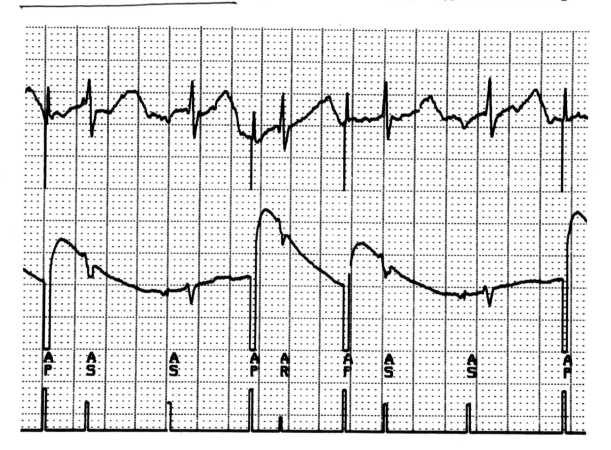

2. There are several ways to correct the far-field sensing problem. The atrial refractory period (ARP) can be lengthened so that the QRS falls within the ARP and is not sensed. Another approach would be to make the atrial sensing circuit less sensitive. If a sensitivity is found where the QRS is no longer sensed by the AAIR pacemaker, the ECG needs to be reassessed to be certain the native atrial events are still being sensed as well.

The AV conduction should be further assessed to determine its stability. This could be accomplished with ambulatory monitoring and/or stress testing.

CASE 4

Question:

Programmed Settings:
Medtronic 7950B

DDD

Lower Rate	50 bpm (1200ms)
Upper Rate	130 bpm (461.5ms)
AV Delay	150 ms (paced); 130ms (sensed)
Rate Adapt AV	ON
PVARP	310 ms
Mode switch	ON
Rate Drop	OFF

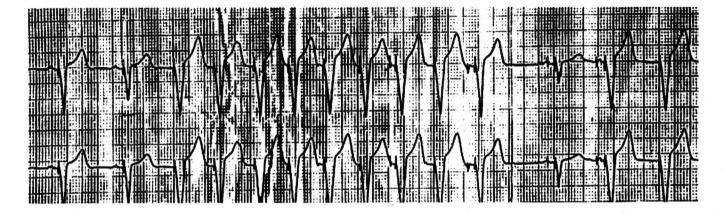

What is the likely cause(s) of the abnormality? Why does the rate change? What accounts for the AV pacing which is observed?

Answer:

Programmed Settings:
Medtronic 7950B
DDD

Lower Rate	50 bpm (1200ms)
Upper Rate	130 bpm (461.5ms)
AV Delay	150 ms (paced); 130 ms (sensed)
Rate Adapt AV	ON
PVARP	310 ms
Mode switch	ON
Rate Drop	OFF

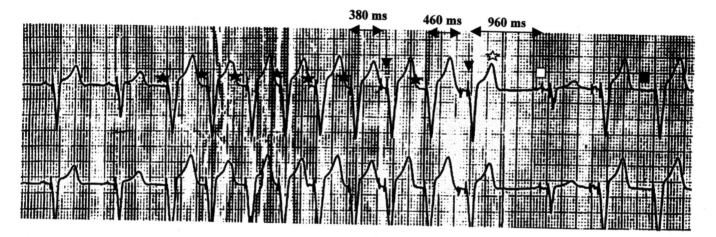

The rapid ventricular paced events are consistent with oversensing in the atrium resulting in tracking (stars indicate atrial sensed events). The arrows indicate AV paced events above the lower rate. When AV pacing above the lower rate occurs one should consider rate drop, rate smoothing, or rate adaptation. Rate drop is not programmed on and usually continues for a longer time. Rate smoothing, pacing in the atrium or the ventricle to maintain the intervals within a certain percentage (3% to 12%) of the preceding intervals, would be a reasonable explanation but is not available in this generator. Thus rate adaptation is the most reasonable explanation. In addition it explains the short AV paced intervals which are due to the rate adaptive AV delay. The long interval of 960 ms may be due to a ventricular sensed event which resets the timing cycle. The last beat on the right represents ventricular pacing, which may be due to tracking in DDD or mode switching to DDIR with atrial oversensing.

CASE 5

Question:

You are presented with the following tracing from a patient in the pacemaker clinic for a routine visit. The patient is rather stoic and initially denies any problems. With further questioning she admits that she occasionally has a very slight and very transient sensation of lightheadedness but had discounted the symptoms. The information you are given is as follows:

Mode:	DDDR
Lower Rate:	50 bpm
Upper rate:	110 bpm
PVARP:	160 ms

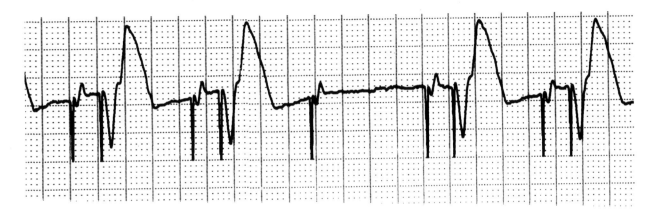

1. List all of the events noted on the tracing.
2. Is pacemaker function normal?
3. Should any programming changes be made?

Answer:

1. The following events occur on the tracing:
   Atrial capture (1)
   Ventricular capture (2)
   Ventricular oversensing (3)

2. Pacemaker function is appropriate for the programmed parameters but is clinically unacceptable with the demonstration of crosstalk. If this were to occur in successive cycles the result would be prolonged ventricular asystole. It is possible that this accounts for the patient's vague symptoms.

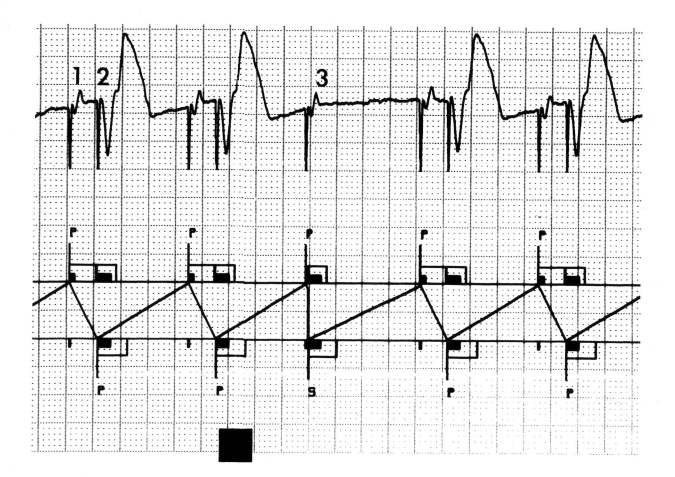

3. If ventricular safety pacing (VSP) is an option it should be turned "on." (Almost all current generation dual-chamber pacemakers have VSP as an option.) There is no clinical reason why VSP should not be activated routinely.

In addition, atrial pacing threshold should be determined and atrial outputs could be decreased if appropriate; and ventricular sensing threshold assessed and ventricular sensitivity be programmed less sensitively if appropriate. Regardless, VSP should be activated.

CASE 6

Question:

A 54-year-old male had a pacemaker implanted 5 years ago for intermittent AV block. At the time of implant acute ventricular thresholds were as follows: 0.5 V, 0.8 mA, 760 Ohms, 12.5 mV R wave. His ventricular lead was placed on medical advisory because of a higher than acceptable incidence of lead insulation failure. He has been on monthly trans-telephonic checks since the advisory was initiated. On the most recent trans-telephonic transmission the following non-magnet tracing was obtained:

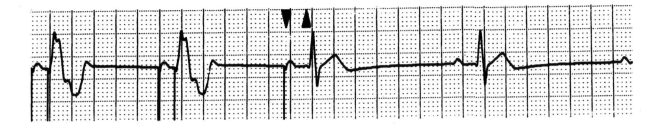

The patient was asymptomatic. You advise the patient to return to the pacemaker clinic. In clinic evaluation reveals intermittent ventricular undersensing and oversensing. The device is not capable of providing telemetered impedance values. A decision is made to proceed with intraoperative troubleshooting. When connected to the PSA the intermittent sensing abnormalities persist. Repetitive impedance measurements are consistently in the range of 500 - 520 Ohms. Chronic ventricular pacing threshold is 1.3 V, 2.7 mA, and R wave of 12 mV.

1. Based on this information what is the most likely diagnosis?
2. Based on the intraoperative measurements, how would you proceed?

Answer:

1. The first two paced complexes occur at the lower rate limit of approximately 50 bpm. Following the 3rd atrial pacing artifact there is no ventricular pacing output. However, the interval to the intrinsically conducted QRS complex appears to be greater than the programmed AV interval that can be measured in the first two complexes. Following this the cycle length between the two intrinsic QRS complexes is significantly greater than 1200 ms or 50 bpm. In this case, the Marker Channel™ fails to recognize the oversensed events, but something must be sensed to result in ventricular output inhibition.

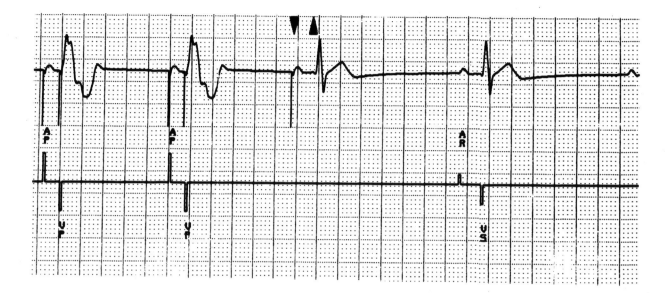

Given the clinical presentation of sensing abnormalities and the known medical advisory, insulation failure would be the most likely etiology. It would be reasonable to obtain a new chest x-ray to assess lead positioning and conductor integrity, but these problems are much less likely than an insulation failure.

2. Insulation failures are classically associated with very low impedance values. Although the reliability of impedance measurements has been a source of controversy, impedance values of 250 Ohms is fairly specific for an insulation failure. There is some literature that suggests a fall in impedance of 30% from the implant impedance value is also suggestive of an insulation failure. In this particular case the impedance value has fallen approximately 30%.

This should be treated as an insulation failure and the lead replaced regardless of the impedance value measured intraoperatively. Impedance values are variable enough that intraoperative measurements should not sway the diagnosis if there are compatible pacing abnormalities and an existing medical advisory.

CASE 7

Question:

An elderly woman is sent for pacing system evaluation. She admits to recent pre-syncopal symptoms. She states that the VVI pacemaker was implanted 8 years ago and it has been more than a year since the pacemaker has been evaluated because she has been preoccupied with her husband's medical care. The pacemaker has only limited telemetric capabilities. In addition to programmed values you learn that the measured lead impedance is 1500 Ohms. No abnormalities are appreciated on the chest x-ray. A segment of her 12-lead ECG is shown here:

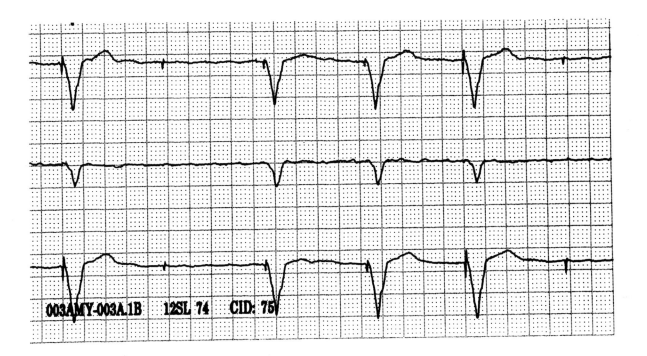

1. How would you proceed? (Note: increasing the voltage amplitude and pulse width to their highest values did not alter the appearance of the ECG.)
2. What is your working differential diagnosis at this point?

Answer:

1. On the previous ECG there is intermittent failure to capture. On the subsequent ECG that is shown below, there is complete failure to capture (**arrows**) and ventricular ectopy. Ventricular sensing still appears to be intact.

Because the failure to capture cannot be correct by reprogramming the output and especially since the patient has been symptomatic, she should be hospitalized until definitive action can be taken.

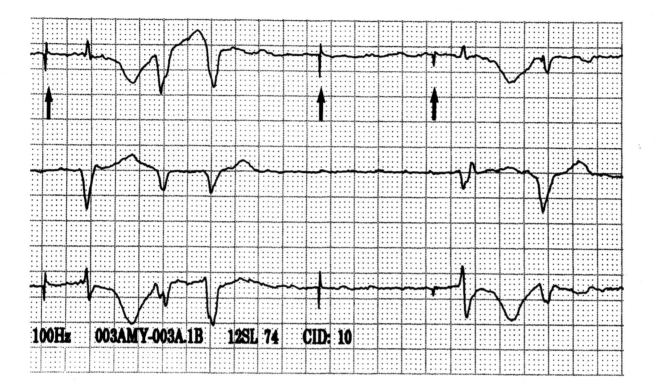

2. The differential diagnosis at this point is quite broad. Failure to capture could represent loss of lead integrity, either insulation failure or conductor fracture, battery depletion, profound exit block, battery depletion, and lead dislodgment. Lead dislodgment at 8 years after implant is unlikely. If there is a lead abnormality, the telemetered impedance value of 1500 Ohms would suggest conductor fracture over lead insulation failure. In a patient with an 8-year-old pacemaker, who appears to be fairly pacemaker dependent, i.e. she may have been pacing the majority of the time, battery depletion is also a viable possibility.

At the time of intraoperative troubleshooting, analysis of the pulse generator demonstrated near complete battery depletion. Repetitive impedance measurements via the PSA were in the 600 to 700 Ohm range. Telemetry values may become less reliable when the battery is so thoroughly depleted. Therefore, the initial impedance value of 1500 Ohms should be dismissed. The chronic lead was connected to a new pacemaker and normal pacing was seen.

CASE 8

Question:

Programmed Settings

DDD
Lower rate   1333 ms (45 bpm)
Upper rate   375 ms(160 bpm)
AV delay   130 ms
PVARP   270 ms
Rate drop   ON
Mode switching   OFF
Rate drop rate   100 bpm

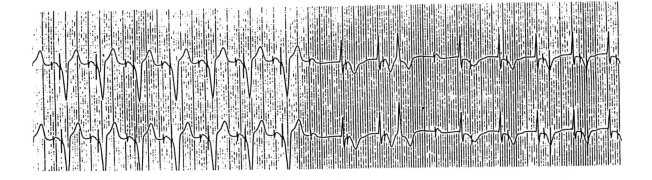

How do you account for the rate at the left of the panel? What causes the change in the rhythm in the right part of the panel?

Answer:

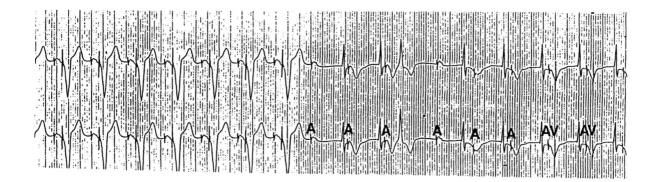

On the left part of the panel, there is evidence of AV pacing at 100 bpm. This is most consistent with rate drop, which is programmed on. In selected pacemaker models, AV pacing at the intervention rate occurs when the atrial rate follows below a programmed value. During rate drop pacing, the mode is still DDD. In the right part of the panel, one sees atrial pacing but not always followed by a ventricular paced event. This is most consistent with ventricular oversensing. The occurrence of the atrial paced events after intrinsic QRS complexes is most consistent with a noise reversion mode.

CASE 9

Question:

A 66-year-old female demonstrates chronotropic incompetence and symptomatic sinus pauses. She also has paroxysmal atrial fibrillation and atrial flutter but her predominant rhythm is sinus. A DDDR pacemaker is implanted and the patient, initially, does well. Shortly after dismissal she calls the pacemaker clinic complaining of increasing difficulties with her tachyarrhythmias. A trans-telephonic tracing is shown:

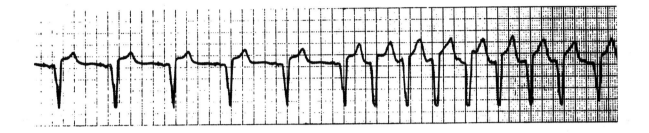

1. How would you explain the transtelephonic tracing?
2. What steps could you take to prevent the symptomatic tachyarrhythmias from reoccurring?

Answer:

1. The transtelephonic tracing is shown below but is now accompanied by a Marker-Channel™ like diagram. The transtelephonic tracing reveals normal sinus rhythm with appropriate ventricular tracking in the initial portion of the tracing. Following this, atrial fibrillation begins and the pacemaker tracks the atrial fibrillation at a rapid rate. (The pacing configuration is bipolar and pacing artifacts are difficult to appreciate. However, all ventricular activity is paced.)

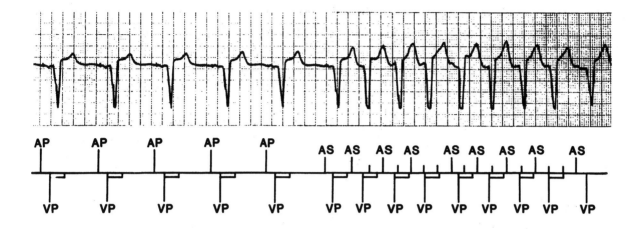

2. This particular DDDR pacemaker did not have mode-switching as a programmable option. Mode-switching is certainly the most appropriate method for managing the paced patient with paroxysmal atrial tachyarrhythmias. In the absence of mode-switching, less satisfactory options are programming to DDIR mode or limiting the maximum tracking rate so that symptoms would be minimized even if the pacemaker was tracking an atrial tachyarrhythmia.

CASE 10

Question:

The Lead II & III recording shown was taken immediately after implantation of a bipolar AAIR pacing system. The atrial lead was in good position and the stimulation and sensing thresholds were within normal limits.

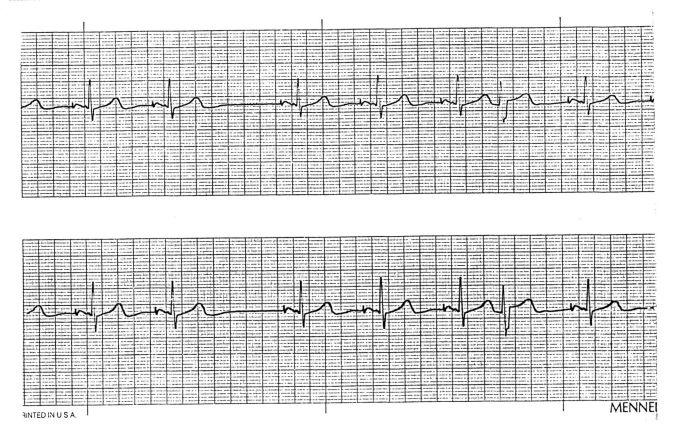

MENNE

What is causing the pause after the second complex?

Answer:

A blocked APB falls on the T wave of the second complex and is sensed and resets the AA timing interval.

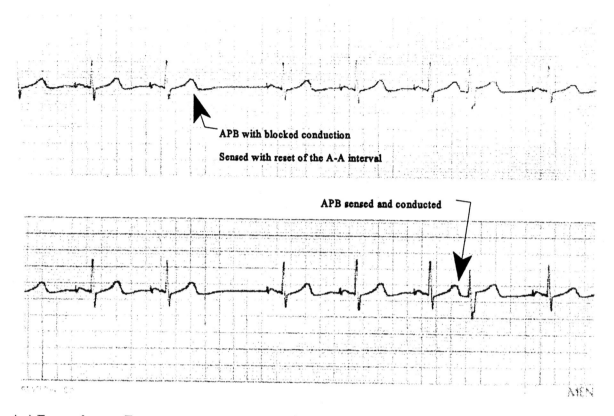

APB with blocked conduction

Sensed with reset of the A-A interval

APB sensed and conducted

AAI pacing ; Lower rate 60 [1000ms], atrial refractory - 450ms

CASE 11

Question:

A 73-year-old physician develops complete heart block following a mitral valve replacement. He has a history of paroxysmal atrial fibrillation. A DDDR pacemaker with mode-switching capabilities is implanted. The following rhythm strip was obtained during routine programming:

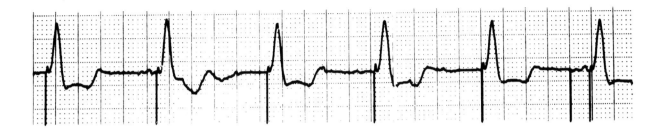

1. Assuming that mode-switching is programmed "on," does the rhythm strip display normal function?
2. In what mode is the pacemaker operating?

Answer:

1. The rhythm strip displays atrial fibrillation and the paced ventricular rate is approximately 50 bpm. Mode-switching is normal.

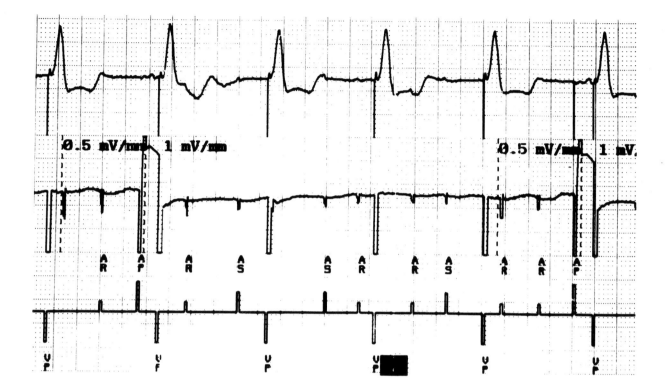

2. Near the end of the rhythm strip, with the patient in atrial fibrillation, AV sequential pacing is seen. The preceding P wave has occurred in the refractory period and is therefore not sensed. This particular pacemaker mode switches to the DDIR mode. This rhythm strip is compatible with DDIR pacing. The atrial pacing artifact was released because the preceding P wave occurred in refractory and in the DDIR mode, an atrial pacing artifact will be delivered if not inhibited by sensed atrial activity.

There is actually atrial pacing earlier in the strip, (see Marker Channel™), but the atrial pacing artifact is not well appreciated on the ECG tracing. This contrasts with the obvious atrial pacing artifact in the last pacing cycle. The difference in the pacing artifact appearance is due to the digital recording system being used. Digital recording systems may result in significant variability in reproduction of the pacing artifacts and the difference in the atrial pacing artifact appearances has no clinical significance.

CASE 12

Question:

Programmed settings:

DDDR
LRL   857 ms (70bpm)
Max. Tracking rate   545 ms (110bpm)
AV Delay   200 ms
PVARP Base*   280 ms

*Shortens as rate increases

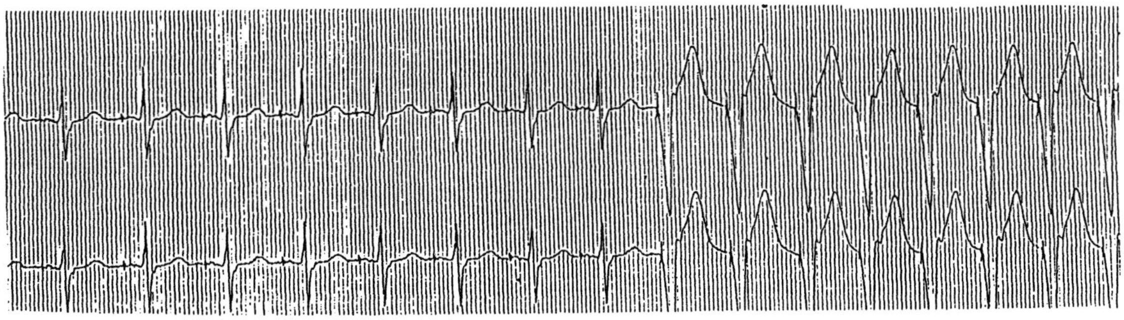

680 ms

600 ms

How do you account for the rhythm on the left part of the panel?
What causes a change on the right part of the panel?

Answer:

At the left panel, there is evidence of atrial pacing at 760 ms cycle length with conduction to the ventricles. Since this is faster than the lower rate, this represents sensor-driven pacing. On the right part of the panel, there is ventricular pacing. Each ventricular paced event is followed by a P wave by about 200 ms. The ventricular pacing is at the upper rate limit (545 ms). Most likely this represents pacemaker-mediated tachycardia. Following each ventricular paced event, the P wave is sensed. The P wave is sensed since the PVARP is shortened due to the sensor-driven rate. The first beat of the pacemaker-mediated tachycardia is initiated by atrial oversensing (1).

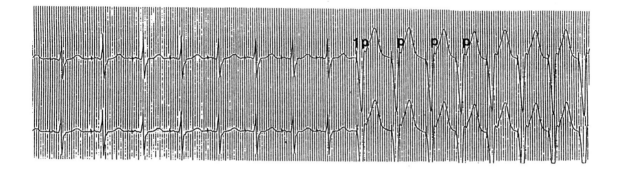

CASE 13

Question:

A 42-year-old female presents elsewhere with recurrent, unprovoked syncope with injury on several occasions. ECG and Holter are normal, as are ventricular stimulation and SNRTs. Tilt-testing results in profound syncope with 9 second pause and fall in BP from 116/78 to 68/32 mm Hg. She is treated with a variety of drugs including beta-blockers, dipyridamole, and ephedrine. She continues to have syncope and returns to her cardiologist who recommends a pacemaker. A VVIR pacemaker is implanted. However, her syncope continues and she complains of increasing malaise. She comes to you for a second opinion.

Her malaise is clearly related to ventricular pacing and you make a diagnosis of pacemaker syndrome. A decision is made to upgrade to a DDD pacemaker. The following ECG tracings were obtained after the pacemaker upgrade and correlated with very mild and transient lightheadedness.

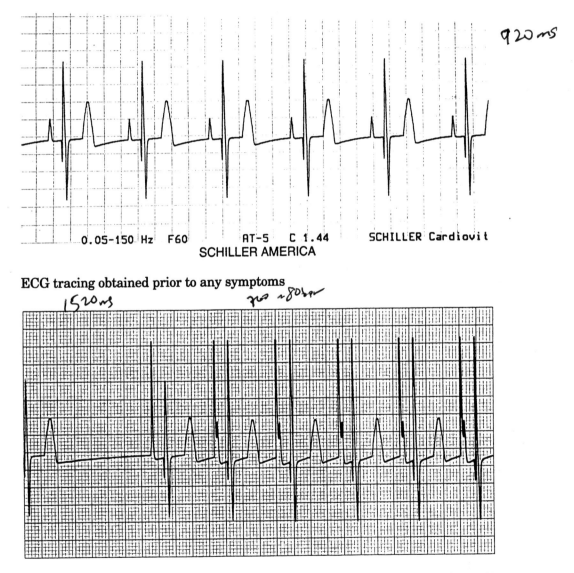

ECG tracing obtained prior to any symptoms

ECG tracing obtained coincident with the mild symptoms

CM721311L.62

1. What is the correct diagnosis?
2. Are the ECG tracings compatible with normal pacemaker function?

Answer:

1. The patient has neurocardiogenic syncope with cardioinhibitory and vasodepressor components. Significant controversy continues regarding optimal treatment for such patients. However, if a permanent pacemaker is used, some definite guidelines exist. Dual-chamber pacing is indicated. Single-chamber atrial pacing is contraindicated because AV block may occur during the episodes. Single-chamber ventricular pacing is suboptimal because pacemaker syndrome may further compound the hypotensive component of the illness and make symptoms worse. The secondary diagnosis in this patient is pacemaker syndrome, secondary to VVIR pacing.

2. The ideal dual-chamber pacemaker would have the capability of faster pacing in response to a sudden change in heart rate. Such features, (e.g. Search Hysteresis™ or Rate Drop Response™), has been shown to have additional benefit in symptom relief in the patient with neurocardiogenic syncope. Upon detection of a sudden rate decrease the pacemaker responds by pacing at a faster rate, i.e. 80 to 100 bpm, for a defined period of time at which point the lower rate or hysteresis rate is resumed.

The first ECG demonstrates normal sinus rhythm with intact ventricular conduction and a rate of approximately 60 bpm. The second ECG begins with a pause followed by AV sequential pacing at approximately 80 bpm. (The heart rate preceding the AV sequential pacing was approximately 40 bpm. This is the electrocardiographic appearance of a feature such as Search Hysteresis™ or Rate Drop Response™.) Hopefully, the faster AV sequential pacing will help support the patient's blood pressure, and thus eliminate or minimize the patient's symptoms.

CASE 14

Question:

A 72-year-old female has a pacemaker implanted for intermittent high-grade AV block. During a routine trans-telephonic transmission at one month post implant, the patient has intermittent ventricular failure to output. The patient is asked to return for further evaluation. Prior to the chest x-ray, the patient is seen in the pacemaker clinic, and the pacemaker thoroughly interrogated. A diagnosis is made based on the in-clinic evaluation. The diagnosis is confirmed by the patient's chest x-ray shown below.

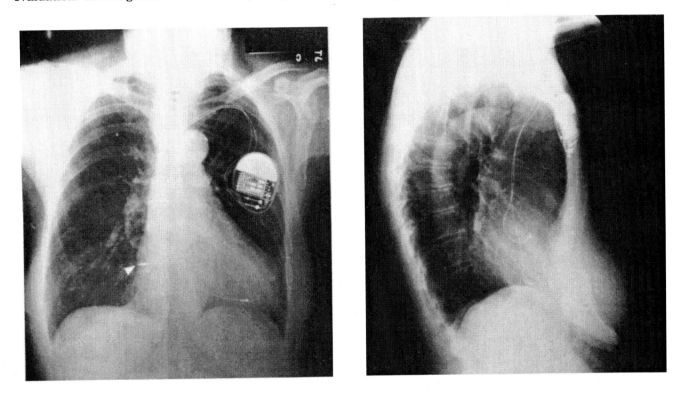

1. Describe the pacing system by trying to detect as many details as possible from the chest x-ray.
2. Can you explain the patient's intermittent ventricular failure to output from the radiographic findings?
3. What is the appropriate treatment?

Answer:

1. The chest x-ray demonstrates a dual-chamber unipolar pacemaker with unipolar atrial and ventricular leads. The pacemaker is placed in a prepectoral position and the leads have most likely been placed via the subclavian vein. Atrial lead position is suboptimal because the "J" is insufficient. (This is pointed out with the arrowhead on the PA film.) It is difficult to follow the entire course of the ventricular lead. The position of the ventricular lead tip is adequate but ideally there would have been more "slack" left in the ventricular lead. Close inspection of the header demonstrates the upper pin, atrial lead, to be completely inserted, and extending beyond connector block. The lower pin, ventricular lead, is not pushed in as far as the upper pin. This is best demonstrated on the close-up view.

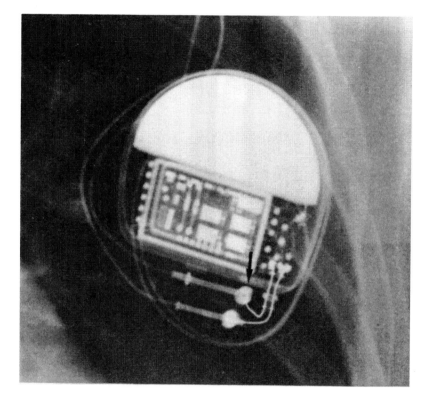

2. As noted in the answer to question 1, there is an abnormal appearance of the connector block. In the close-up radiograph provided it should be recognized that one of the connector pins is not completely through the connector block. Presumably the lead was not adequately secured in the connector block at the time of implant. Intermittent contact allowed only intermittent failure to output.

3. The only way to correct the problem is to re-open the pacemaker pocket and adequately secure the lead in the connector block.

CASE 15

Question:

A 58-year-old female presents with near syncope. Ambulatory monitoring reveals marked chronotropic incompetence and sinus pauses. There is no evidence of AV node dysfunction. An AAIR pacemaker is implanted. Initial follow-up is unremarkable. At approximately 1 year following pacemaker implantation the patient returns with nonspecific complaints of general malaise, mild to moderate exercise intolerance, and vague chest discomfort. An echocardiogram reveals normal left ventricular function and resting 12 lead ECG demonstrates normal AAI pacing at the programmed lower rate limit of 60 bpm. An exercise test is performed. The following tracing is obtained during the exercise test:

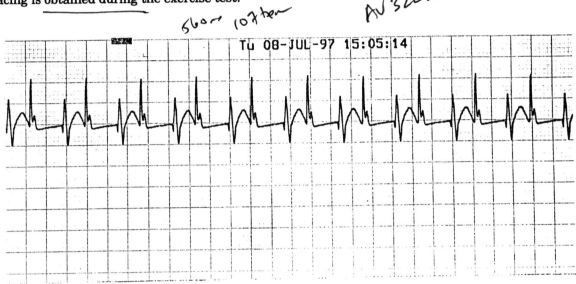

1. Is the ECG tracing normal?
2. What is your diagnosis?
3. How would you proceed?

Answer:

1. The ECG tracing reveals rate-adaptive atrial pacing at a rate of 110 bpm. The upper rate limit was programmed to 120 bpm so the patient had not yet reached this limit. Note that the AR interval is approximately 320 ms.

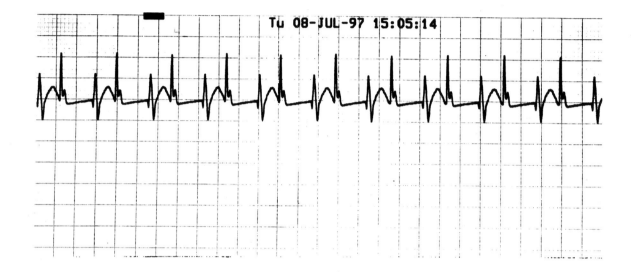

2. The history provided states that AV node function was felt to be normal at the time of pacemaker implantation but there is no mention of whether incremental atrial pacing was performed at the time of atrial pacemaker implantation. Accepted protocol would be to demonstrate 1:1 AV conduction up to paced atrial rates of 120 to 140 bpm. It is not possible to say if AV conduction was abnormal at the time of the procedure or whether it has developed in the interim. Regardless, AV node function is not normal at this time. The excessively long AR interval has effectively dissociated AV synchrony. The atrial pacing artifact at the faster sensor-driven rate is occurring closer to the preceding QRS complex than the following QRS complex. The patient has developed pacemaker syndrome. Although classically associated with ventricular pacing, pacemaker syndrome can occur with any mode if effective AV dissociation occurs.

3. The patient needs to be upgraded to a dual-chamber pacemaker, i.e. a ventricular lead should be placed. The AV interval should be programmed to a physiologic interval. Because the patient is active and capable of achieving faster paced rates, she may also benefit from a rate-adaptive AV interval.

CASE 16

Question:

A patient with a DDDR pacemaker placed for sinus node dysfunction presents for routine pacemaker evaluation. The pacemaker is programmed to a lower rate of 70 bpm and upper rate of 120 bpm. The patient is rarely aware of "heart racing" and an event recorder is used to try and capture the rare episodes. The patient called to report that an episode had occurred while she was resting and she transmitted the recording. The terminal portion of the episode is shown:

520 ~ 116ppm

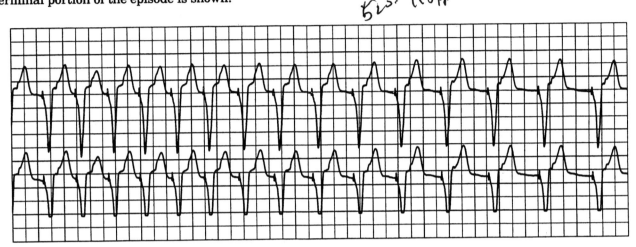

CM174843.10

1. How would you interpret this electrocardiographic tracing?
2. Are there any other clinical issues that should be addressed relative to this episode?

100% V-pace.
No atrial p—
Retrograde p-wave.

Answer:

1. The ECG is compatible with mode switching. Although it is not possible to identify the atrial activity, the tracing begins with ventricular tracking at a rate of approximately 120 bpm, the programmed upper rate limit. The rate then gradually slows to approximately 70 bpm at the end of the tracing. Since the patient reported that she was at rest at the time of the episode, it is likely that after mode switching, the pacemaker would have slowed to a rate at or near the lower rate limit.

2. If the pacemaker has a mode-switch counter, it would be reasonable to review this stored information to assess how often the patient was having the paroxysmal supraventricular rhythm disturbance. If they are well tolerated, thanks to the mode-switching, then no specific therapy may be necessary. If the arrhythmia is atrial flutter or atrial fibrillation, the patient's anticoagulation status should be reviewed.

CASE 17

Question:

You are presented with the following tracing from a patient in the pacemaker clinic for a routine visit. The patient is not pacemaker dependent and is asymptomatic. The information you are given is as follows:

Mode:	DDDR
Lower Rate:	70 bpm
Upper Rate:	120 bpm
AV Interval:	200 ms
Voltage amplitude:	5.0 V in both chambers
Pulse width:	0.5 ms in both chambers

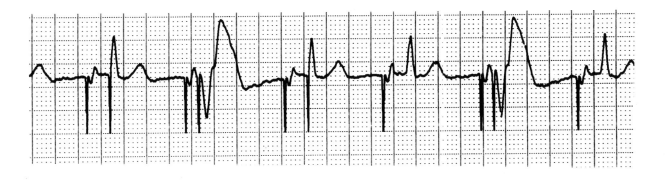

1. List all of the events noted on the tracing.
2. Is pacemaker function normal?
3. Should any programming changes be made?

atrial pacing
ventricular pacing
pseudo fusion
Ventricular sensing
Safety pacing

↓ Ventricle sensitivity
or
↑ VB period
↑ AV del

Answer:

1. The following events occur on the tracing:
   Atrial capture (**1**)
   Ventricular pseudofusion (**2**)
   Ventricular capture (3)
   Ventricular safety pacing (VSP) (**4**)
   Appropriate ventricular inhibition by intrinsic QRS (**5**)

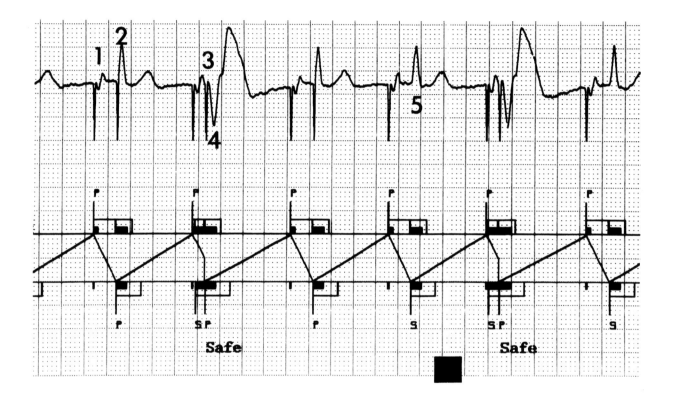

2. The pacemaker is functioning appropriately even though an abnormal interaction between the atrial and ventricular chambers is occurring. With the help of the Marker Channel™ can you identify the cause of the VSP?
   In the two cycles where VSP occurs, look carefully at the ventricular channel of the Marker Channel™. There is initially a sensed event on the ventricular channel (**S**) that occurs almost immediately after the paced atrial event. This is following by a paced ventricular event (**P**) approximately 100 ms later. The initial sensed event (**S**) is crosstalk, i.e. the ventricular sensing circuit is sensing the atrial pacing output. This is sensed after the blanking period and during the cross-talk sensing window resulting in VSP.

3. There are no safety issues with the pacemaker programmed to the current values because even though there is crosstalk, VSP prevents ventricular asystole. However, the crosstalk could possibly be avoided by decreasing the atrial output. This should only be done after atrial pacing thresholds are checked and it is determined that atrial outputs could be decreased and still maintain an adequate pacing margin.

CASE 18

Question:

You are presented with the following tracing from a patient in the pacemaker clinic for a routine visit. The patient is asymptomatic. The information you are given is as follows:

Mode: DDD
Lower Rate: 50 bpm
Upper rate: 110 bpm
PVARP: 250 ms

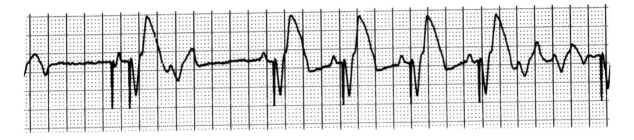

1. List all of the events noted on the tracing.
2. Is pacemaker function normal?
3. What is the atrial rate and what is the ventricular rate?

atrial pacing
ventricular pacing
atrial sensing 75

Answer:

1. The following events occur on the tracing:
   Atrial capture (**1**)
   Ventricular capture (**2**)
   Appropriate atrial sensing (**3**)
   Appropriate ventricular sensing (**4**)

2. Pacemaker function appears normal with P-synchronous pacing at a rate of approximately 77 bpm, appropriately sensed PVCs, and a single cycle with AV sequential pacing.

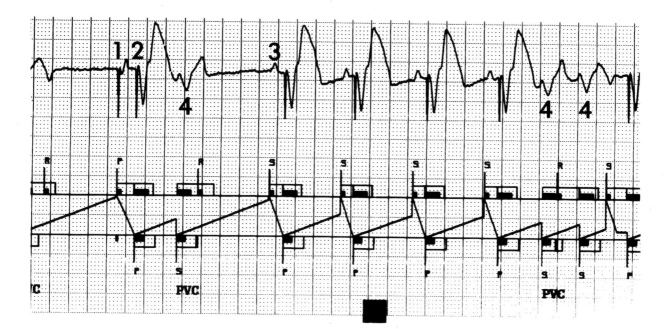

3. The pacemaker appropriately identifies the PVCs. (The pacemaker definition of a PVC is when 2 consecutive ventricular events occur without an intervening atrial event.)

CASE 19

Question:

Vera was implanted 5 years ago with a bipolar DDDR pacing system for Sinus Node Dysfunction. She presented to the pacemaker clinic with complaints of pre-syncope.

The programmed parameters are:

DDD at low-rate 70, AVI-140ms, atrial and ventricular outputs 2.5v at 0.4ms.

MAGNET CANCELLED

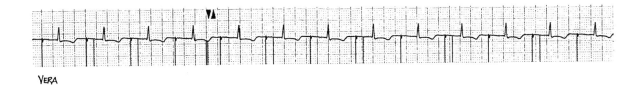

VERA

What is the most likely explanation for the absent ventricular stimulus output?

What is the most likely explanation for the narrow QRS.?

Ventric Non-capture

ventra Non-output

? V- oversensing

atrial capture

long intrinsic AVD

Answer:

The rhythm strip "A," with simultaneous timing diagram and electrogram shown below, was recorded while recumbent. Rhythm strip "B" with simultaneous timing diagram and electrogram was taken while sitting and during deep breathing.

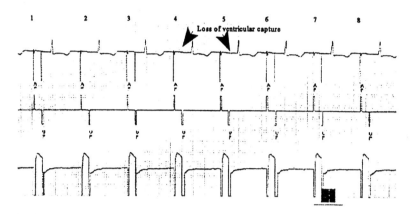

Strip A [Vera]

In the 2,4,5, and 8th complex the ventricular output stimulus is initiated as seen on the timing diagram but is absent on the surface ECG.

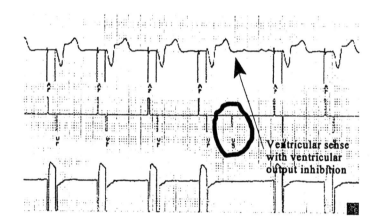

Strip B [Vera]

While sitting and deep breathing ventricular capture is maintained and an episode of inappropriate ventricular inhibition [oversensing] is seen after the 4th complex.

Rhythm strip ('A') shows consistent atrial capture with loss of ventricular capture. After review of the timing diagram 'marker' recording taken simultaneously with the surface ECG, it is evident that the ventricular stimulus is present but does not initiate ventricular capture.

With further review it was noted that while sitting, ventricular capture was maintained, however, periods of ventricular inhibition [oversensing] were observed.

Final interpretation: Bipolar ventricular lead insulation failure presenting with loss of ventricular capture and inappropriate ventricular inhibition [oversensing].

CASE 20

Question:

You are presented with the following tracing from a patient in the pacemaker clinic for an unscheduled visit. The patient complains of transient episodes of lightheadedness and intermittent awareness of a rapid heart rate. The patient is pacemaker dependent. The information you are given is as follows:

Mode:	DDD
Lower Rate:	60 bpm
Upper rate:	115 bpm
Sensed AV interval:	140 ms
Paced AV interval:	160 ms
PVARP:	200 ms

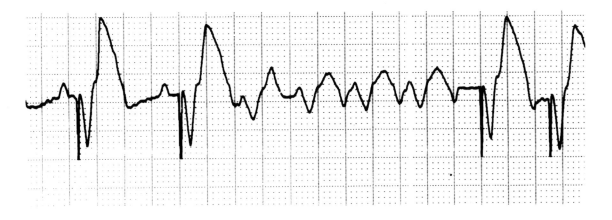

1. List all of the events noted on the tracing.
2. Is pacemaker function normal?
3. Should any programming changes be made?

atrial sense
V- pace
V sense
PVC'n
tracking @ upper rate
PmT
↑ PVARP

Answer:

30. Timing Cycles

1. The following events occur on the tracing:

                    Appropriate atrial sensing (**1**)
                    Ventricular capture (**2**)
                    Ventricular ectopy (**3**)
                    Appropriate ventricular sensing (**3**)
                    Sensed retrograde P wave (**4**)
                    Onset of pacemaker mediated tachycardia (**5**)

2. Pacemaker function is normal.

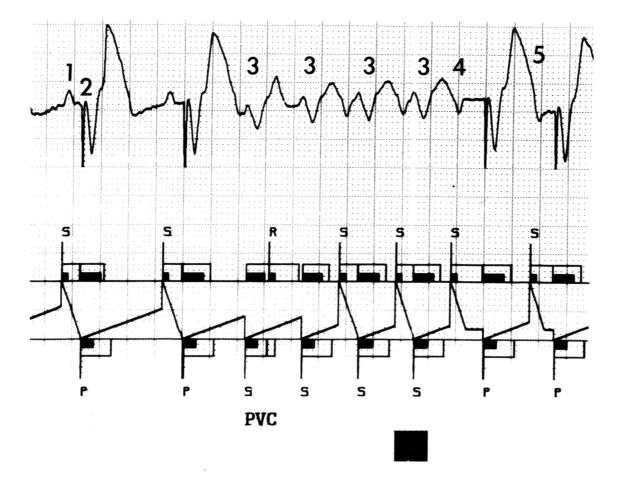

3. Programming changes should be made to prevent the pacemaker mediated tachycardia. There are potentially several options. If the pacemaker has a programmable PMT algorithm, this could be activated, PVARP extension after PVC could be programmed "on," or the PVARP lengthened. With a sensed AV of 140 ms and a desired upper rate limit of 115 bpm, 521 ms, the PVARP could be lengthened without compromising the desired upper rate limit. Currently the TARP = 140 + 200 = 340 ms. Therefore, the PVARP could be lengthened significantly and still allow an upper rate limit of 115 bpm.

    The tracing demonstrates 4 consecutive ventricular events that appear to be ectopic. Given the patient's symptoms of transient lightheadedness there would some concern that the symptoms could be secondary to ventricular arrhythmias. Further evaluation should be pursued.

CASE 21

Question:

A 68-year-old woman has a pacemaker implanted for sinus node dysfunction. She is referred to you 13 months after pacemaker implantation after presenting with a cerebrovascular accident. She is left with only a minor neurological deficit after her CVA. Her PA and lateral chest x-ray is shown below:

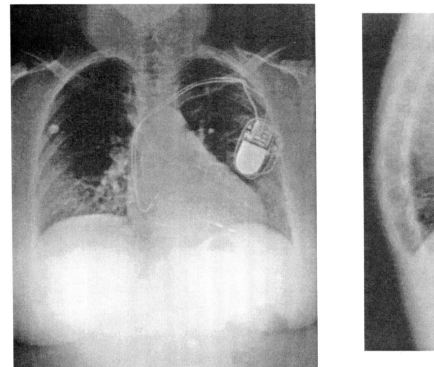 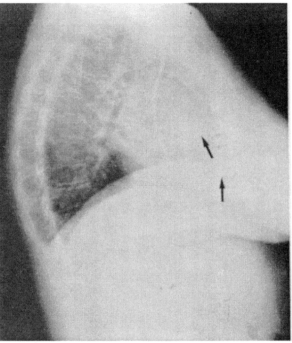

PH723239_2.DIG

1. Describe the pacing system by trying to detect as many details as possible from the chest x-ray.
2. Is there any clue from the chest x-ray regarding the etiology of the patient's recent CVA?
3. What therapeutic advice would you offer?

① Axillary vein approach - acute
  or ?
② PPM generator ② sub pectoral
③ Bipolar atrial lead
  — RAA
④ Bipolar V-lead RV apex

Answer:

1. The chest x-ray demonstrates a dual-chamber pacemaker with two bipolar leads. The pacemaker is placed in the left pre-pectoral position. There is a sharp angle at the point where the leads appear to enter the vascular tree. The atrial lead appears to be appropriately positioned, probably in the right atrial appendage. The ventricular lead turns toward the left chest at a very high point, i.e. above the right atrial lead. The ventricular lead position would normally follow the course of the atrial lead and cross the tricuspid valve at some point near the bottom of the atrial "J" lead or lower.

On the lateral film the lead tips are marked with "arrows." Note that the ventricular lead tip is posterior, not anterior, as would be expected with right ventricular apical positioning.

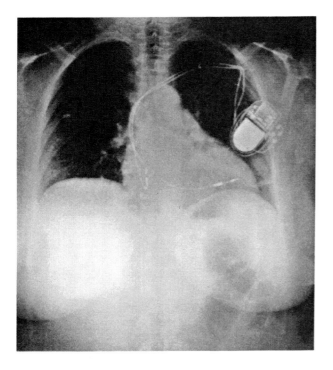
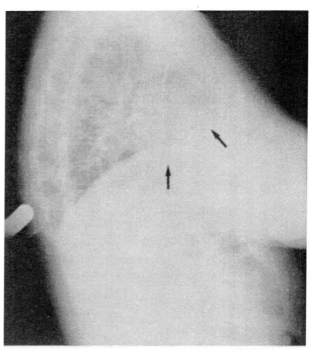

PH723239_1.DIG

2. As noted in the answer to question 1, there is an unusual course of the ventricular lead on the PA film in that it has a higher "take-off" from the right atrium than would normally be expected. This is confirmed in the lateral chest x-ray by the posterior position of the ventricular lead. The combination of these findings confirms the placement of the ventricular transvenous lead in the left ventricle. Anytime a lead is placed in the systemic circulation, or whenever there is right-to-left shunting in a patient with normally placed transvenous pacing system, the patient is at a relatively high-risk for embolization to the central arterial circulation resulting in TIA or CVA.

3. If left ventricular lead placement had been recognized within a matter of hours or even one or two days, it would be reasonable to percutaneously withdraw the lead and reposition in the right ventricle. This patient has had the lead in place for 13 months and already experienced an embolic event with the assumption that the pacing lead was the source of emboli. Percutaneous lead extraction would carry an extremely high risk of further embolic events at the time of the procedure. The only therapeutic options would be to chronically anticoagulate the patient with warfarin or remove the lead during an open heart procedure.

CASE 22

Question:

Marianne, a 47-year-old woman was implanted with a VDD pacing system for complete AV block. Two days after successful device implantation, Marianne experienced prepacing symptoms of pre-syncope. The programmed parameters are VDD with a low rate of 40 bpm and AV interval of 150ms. Ambulatory monitoring is shown.

atrial rate 88
V - V-2   37.5

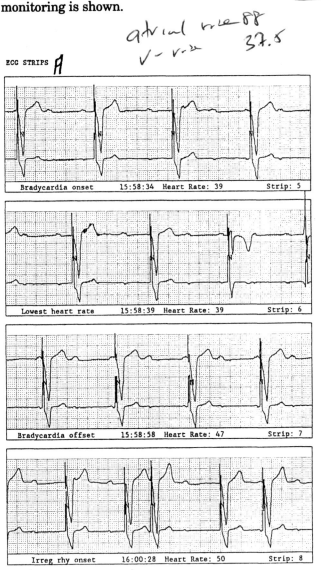

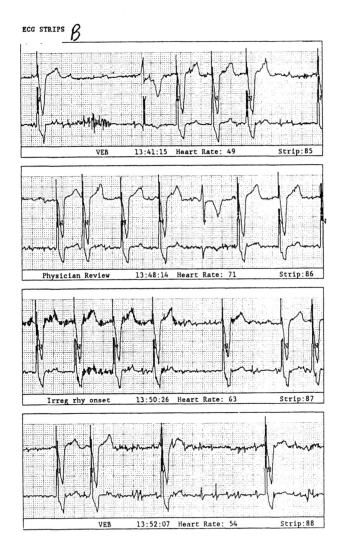

Is atrial and ventricular sensing normal?

Answer:

The holter recording shows loss of atrial sensing with the low rate of 40 [functional VVI pacing] in rhythm strip 'A'. In strip 'B,' during walking, there is an intermittent loss of atrial sensing with episodes of ventricular inhibition due to myopotential sensing. This device operates in a **Unipolar** pacing and sensing configuration.

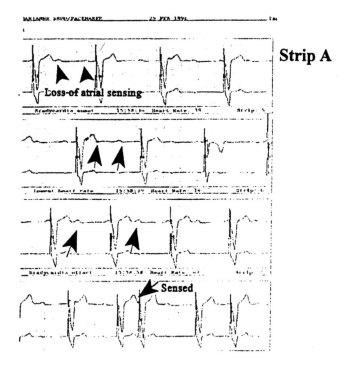

Strip A

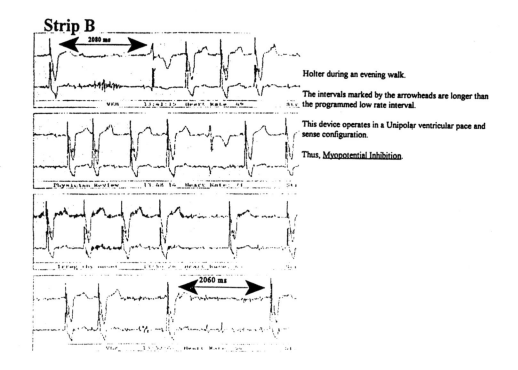

Strip B

Holter during an evening walk.

The intervals marked by the arrowheads are longer than the programmed low rate interval.

This device operates in a Unipolar ventricular pace and sense configuration.

Thus, Myopotential Inhibition.

Final interpretation: Loss of atrial sensing as well as myopotential inhibition of the ventricular channel.

CASE 23

Question:

You are presented with the following tracing from a patient in the pacemaker clinic for a visit prompted by a conversation during a preceding trans-telephonic evaluation. The pacemaker had been implanted 3 months earlier for sinus node dysfunction and AV block. In recent weeks he has had intermittent malaise and also notes intermittent "pounding in his neck." He also states that he remembers being told that his pulse rate should not be less than 70 bpm and believes that his pulse has been slightly less than 70 bpm. He is quick to add that he's not very confident about his ability to check his pulse. The information you are given is as follows:

Mode:	DDDR
Lower Rate:	70 bpm
Upper rate:	120 bpm
Sensed AV interval:	160 ms
Paced AV interval:	200 ms
PVARP:	300 ms

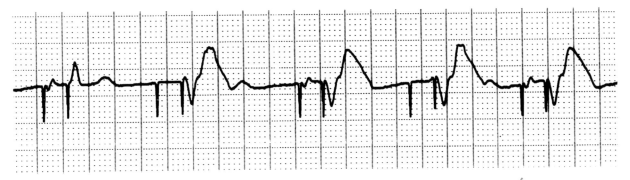

1. List all of the events noted on the tracing.
2. Is pacemaker function normal?
3. Should any programming changes be made?

atrial pacing / capture
V- pacing / capture
Ventricular pseudo fusion
atrial NON-capture
retrograde P-waves

↑ atrial output
Change AV delay

Answer:

1. The following events occur on the tracing:
>   Intermittent atrial capture (**1**)
>   Ventricular fusion or pseudofusion (**2**)
>   Intermittent atrial failure to (**3**)
>   Ventricular capture (**4**)
>   Ventricular oversensing (**5**)
>   Far-field sensing on the atrial channel (**6**)

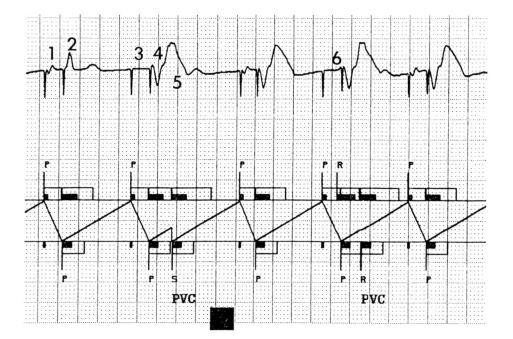

2. Pacemaker function is abnormal. Where the timing diagram notes "PVC" there is a sensed ventricular event (**S**) that follows a paced ventricular event (**P**). This coincides with the T wave which appears to be intermittently sensed on the ventricular sensing channel. This event resets ventricular timing and results in a ventricular cycle length, 1100 ms , that is longer than the programmed lower rate limit of 850 ms. If this happened repetitively it could explain the slower pulse rate to which the patient referred. The T wave oversensing is designated as a PVC because the pacemaker's definition of a PVC is the occurrence of 2 successive ventricular events without an intervening atrial event.

There is also intermittent atrial failure to capture. There are consistent atrial pacing artifacts but inspection of the surface tracing reveals intermittent atrial depolarization. It would be ideal to have another lead to confirm the lack of atrial depolarization but this single tracing is highly suggestive. If the atrial failure to capture is at times consistent, the loss of AV syncope could create pacemaker syndrome, and account for the patient's symptoms of malaise and prominent pulsations in his neck.

There is also oversensing on the atrial channel. At (6), inspection of the timing diagram demonstrates a sensed atrial event (P) followed by an event on the atrial channel designated as (R) or refractory. It is not clear what is being sensed at this point.

3. Atrial pacing thresholds should be determined and outputs increased to see if consistent atrial capture can be maintained. The reason for intermittent atrial failure to capture should also be pursued, i.e. lead dislodgment, exit block, loss of lead integrity.

To avoid T wave oversensing, after determining ventricular sensing threshold, the ventricular sensitivity could be made less sensitive. The ventricular refractory period (VRP) could also be lengthened. Although not stated in the initial information provided, it appears from the timing diagram that the VRP is approximately 220 ms.

CASE 24

Question:

Programmed settings

DDD
LRL   1000 ms (60 bpm)
URL   600 ms (100bpm)
AV delay   140 ms
PVARP   280 ms
V amplitude 5V
V pulse width 0.5 ms

In the top line of the figure below, the rhythm without magnet is shown. The magnet is then applied. How do you account for the observed changes?

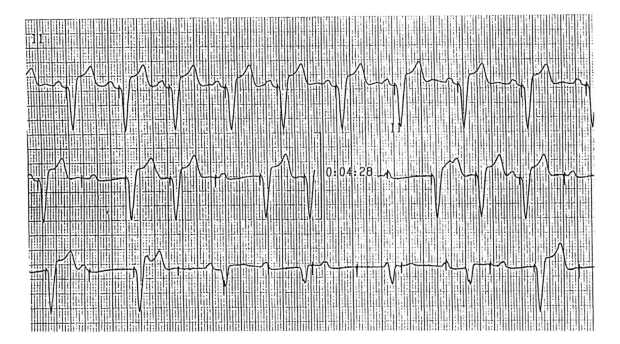

Answer:

There is evidence of ventricular pacing at 100 bpm initiated by the magnet. This pacemaker's magnet mode must be VOO rather than DOO even though the programmed mode is DDD. The failure to sense the intrinsic QRS complexes is consistent with the VOO mode. The ventricular spikes only intermittently capture. Why is this? In the top panel, ventricular pacing occurs with atrial tracking at cycle lengths between 680 ms and 900 ms. However, ventricular pacing occurs at about 600 ms.

It is appealing to think that the output changes with application of magnet. However, continuous decrease in pacing amplitude does not occur in any generator. Only a decrease in output for several beats is available in some generators upon magnet application as part of a threshold margin test. At 100 bpm, the pacing threshold was 1.0 ms at 5 V. Since the generator had been left at the nominal setting of 5 V and 0.5 ms, there was intermittent failure to capture. In contrast, at 60 bpm, the ventricular threshold was 0.375 ms at 5 V. This explains why at baseline without magnet application, 100% capture was seen.

This is an unusual example of rate-dependent pacing thresholds.

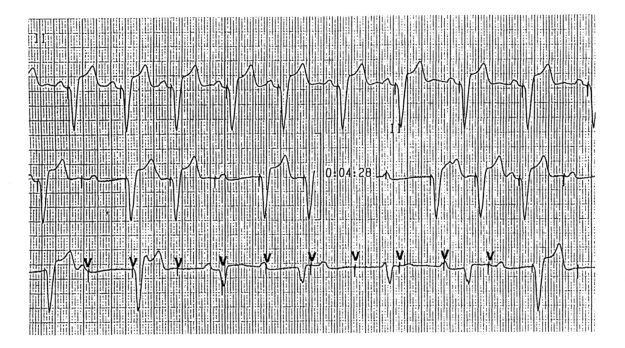

CASE 25

Question:

Called to the ER to see a 20-year-old male admitted emergently with hypotension and diagnosed with cardiac tamponade. You had implanted a permanent pacing system 18 months earlier. The tamponade is successfully managed and you are asked to assess the pacing system and whether it played a role in the tamponade. A PA and lateral chest x-ray obtained after the tamponade was successfully treated is shown below

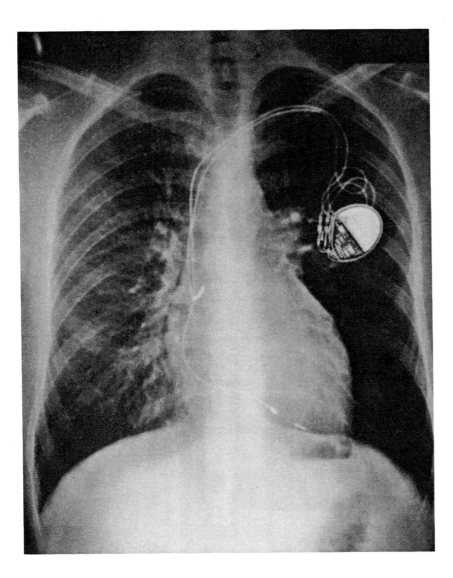

1. Does the chest x-ray help in explaining the tamponade?
2. What steps should be taken in the patient's subsequent management?

Answer:

1. On initial inspection of the PA chest x-ray, the pacing system appears normal. It is a dual-chamber bipolar pacemaker connected to bipolar atrial and ventricular leads. The pacemaker is in a prepectoral position, the leads appear to have been placed via the subclavian vein, and intracardiac lead positioning of both leads appear adequate.

Although difficult to appreciate even when inspecting the actual film, there is an abnormality associated with the atrial lead. A small wire is protruding from the distal aspect of the atrial lead. This lead, the Telectronics Accufix™ lead, was placed on medical advisory after several episodes of J-wire retention fracture. This is a small wire located just under the insulation and separate from the conductor coil that maintains the "J" shape of the lead. If the retention wire breaks and protrudes through the insulation laceration of the heart or great vessels can occur. (See close-up.)

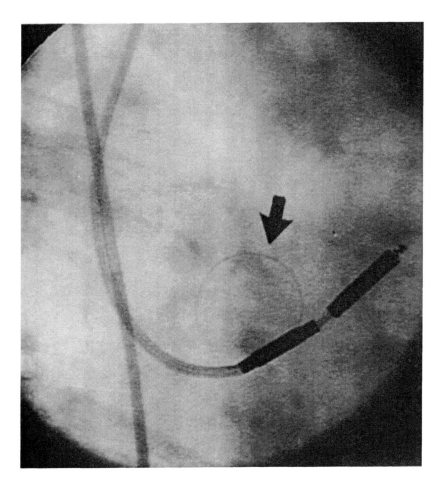

2. In cases where the retention wire has broken and is protruding through the insulation, the lead should be extracted. Individual patient counseling should decide management if the lead is fluoroscopically normal or if the wire is fractured but not extruded through the insulation.

CASE 26

Question:

A 55-year-old male receives a DDDR pacemaker for AV block. He also has mild chronotropic incompetence. Acute pacing thresholds are excellent. The pacemaker is programmed to the following parameters:

Mode:	DDDR
Lower rate:	60 bpm
Upper rate:	100 bpm
AV delay:	175 ms
PVARP:	250 ms

The following non-magnet ECG tracing is obtained during his first pacemaker follow-up.

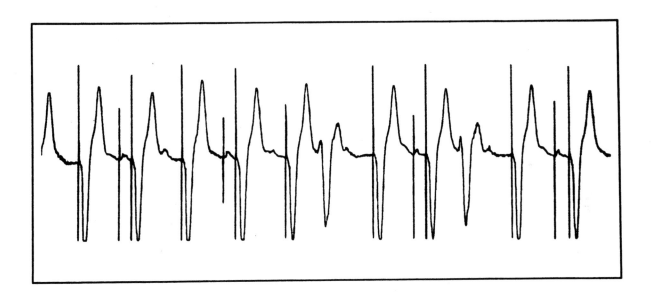

1. Does the ECG tracing reflect appropriate function given the patient's programmed parameters?
2. Are any programming changes required?

atrial capture
V- capture
intrinsic atrial/sense
V- sense

Answer:

1. Pacemaker function is normal and compatible with programmed parameters. A DDDR pacemaker must abide by DDD timing cycles as well as display appropriate rate-adaptive function. In this tracing, the ventricular cycle length varies from 600 ms to 630 ms. The shorter ventricular cycles emerge with AV sequential pacing. By definition, AV sequential pacing at any rate greater than the programmed lower rate must be sensor-driven. The slightly longer ventricular cycles are driven by a sinus beat. However, notice that the PV intervals vary and that the VV interval of the sinus-driven cycles are all at 600 ms which is also the maximum tracking rate. The pacemaker cannot track at rates greater than the effective maximum tracking rate and therefore pseudo-Wenckebach behavior is seen. The slightly longer sensor-driven cycles reflect rate-adaptive sensor programming. In this example, there is very little difference in the sensor-driven and sinus-driven cycle lengths. This reflects reasonable rate-adaptive programming.

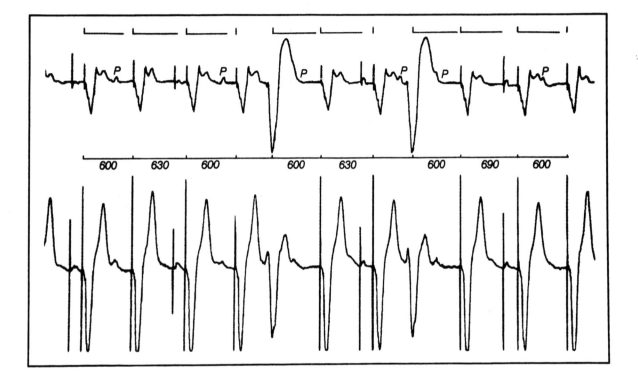

2. No programming changes are required unless it is determined clinically that the patient should be allowed a faster maximum tracking rate.

CASE 27

Question:

David was implanted three years ago with a bipolar DDDR pacing system for combined Sinus Node Dysfunction and Atrioventricular block. Six months ago his follow-up assessment was normal; showing normal pulse generator telemetry data, nominal lead performance, and normal stimulation threshold of the ventricle. However, due to persistent atrial fibrillation David was reprogrammed from DDD to VVIR. Stimulation thresholds on all previous clinic assessments were below 1.0 volts. David presented to his family physician with new onset signs of congestive failure.

The 12 lead ECG and pacemaker telemetry data shown was taken on presentation to the clinic.

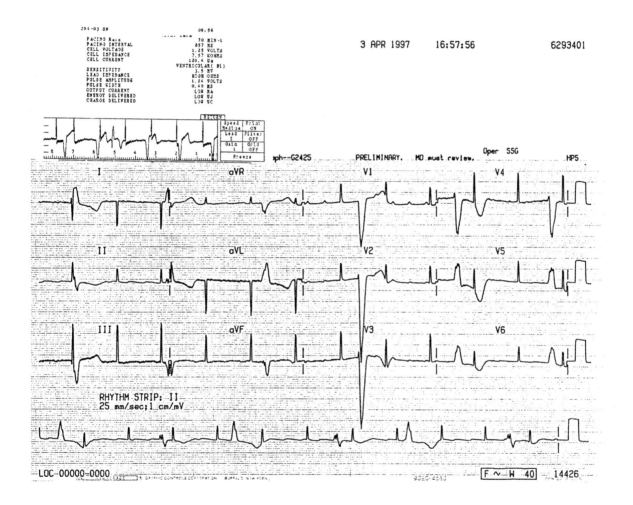

What is the most likely cause for the loss of ventricular capture?

Answer:

With an increase in ventricular output from 3.5 volts to 5.0 volts and 1.0 ms, loss of ventricular capture was still evident. The battery telemetry data reveals that the voltage output has decreased to 1.24 volts and is sub-threshold for this patient, thus sustained loss of ventricular capture occurs. The initial concern with respect to the lead telemetry was the recorded "HIGH" ohms.

During surgical intervention the ventricular lead tested within optimal limits. **Due to the extreme drop in battery cell voltage all other telemetry data are inaccurate.**

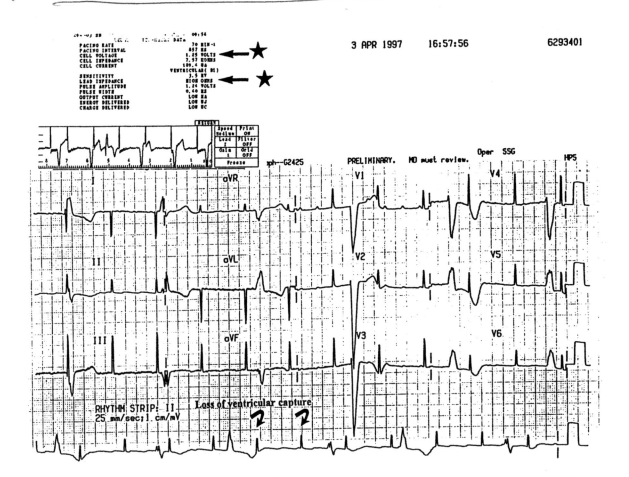

Final interpretation: Premature battery depletion with output delivery at sub-threshold with subsequent sustained loss of ventricular capture.

CASE 28

Question:

A 70-year-old female receives a VVI pacemaker for rare episodes of AV block. The patient has no history of ventricular or supraventricular rhythm disturbances. The implant is uncomplicated and acute thresholds are excellent. Occasional PVCs are noted during lead placement. The pacemaker is programmed to VVI at 50 bpm. Several hours after the patient returns to her room you are called by her nurse who reports significant extrasystoles. The nurse is requesting an order for intravenous lidocaine. The patient is asymptomatic. An ECG tracing representative of the nurse's observations is shown here:

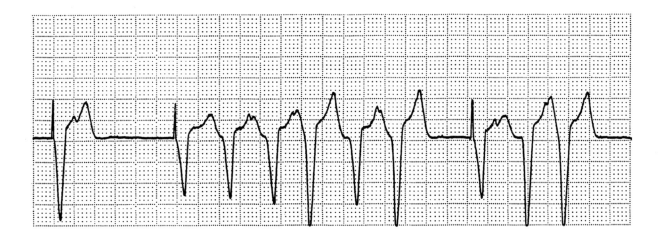

CM175867L.01

1. How would you interpret the ECG tracing?
2. How would you treat the ECG findings?

Answer:

1. The ECG reveals three paced complexes with some variation in the paced QRS morphology suggesting that one of the morphologies probably represents a fusion beat. Although it is impossible to be certain from this ECG tracing alone, the second and third paced events probably represent the paced QRS morphology and the first event likely represents fusion with a true PVC. There are 5 ventricular complexes that occur between the 2nd and 3rd paced events. Three of these 5 events are of identical morphology to the paced QRS morphology (**asterisk**). The complexes labeled with arrows are probably PVCs and note that the presumed PVC that precedes the 3rd paced event is not sensed. Measuring back from the 3rd paced event by 1200 ms, 50 bpm, coincides with a complex of similar morphology to the paced events.

This rhythm strip demonstrates:

VVI pacing
"Tip" extrasystoles (repetitive beating after a paced ventricular event that is of similar morphology to the paced QRS morphology)
PVCs
Failure to sense what is presumed to be a PVC (**second arrow**)

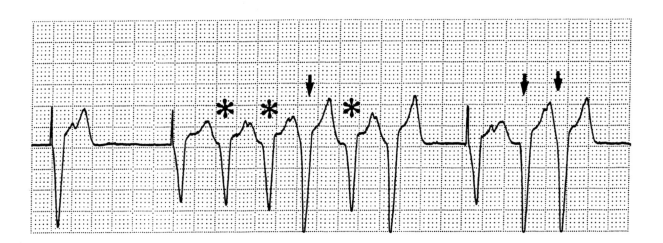

CM175867L.01

2. "Tip" extrasystoles generally do not require treatment. Although lidocaine or a similar antiarrhythmic may decrease their frequency, left untreated they will usually stop within 24 hours following lead placement. This patient is complicated by the fact that there are probably some true PVCs. However, ventricular rhythm disturbances have never been a clinical problem for this patient and it's possible that this second morphology of extrasystoles may also stop spontaneously. In this actual case, the patient was simply observed. By the next morning, only rare PVCs were seen and the patient remained asymptomatic.

Failure to sense a PVC is not uncommon either early or late after pacemaker implantation. When intraoperative sensing thresholds are checked, one is measuring the intrinsic R wave as seen from the vector of the lead. Since a PVC can occur from anywhere in the ventricle, and the vector may be significantly different than that of the intrinsic QRS complex, it is not surprising that the PVC may not be seen as being of sufficient amplitude for sensing. It is reasonable to reprogram the sensitivity to a more sensitive value in an attempt to sense the PVCs. If this is unsuccessful, and if this is a rare occurrence and sensing is otherwise normal, it is probably safe to observe.

CASE 29

Question:

You are presented with the following tracing from a patient in the pacemaker clinic for a routine visit.
The patient is pacemaker dependent and notes intermittent awareness of a faster heart rate while he is at rest.
The information you are given is as follows:

Mode: DDD
Lower Rate: 60 bpm
Upper rate: 95 bpm
Sensed AV interval: 200 ms
Paced AV interval: 200 ms
PVARP: 150 ms

600ml → Hn 100 bpm

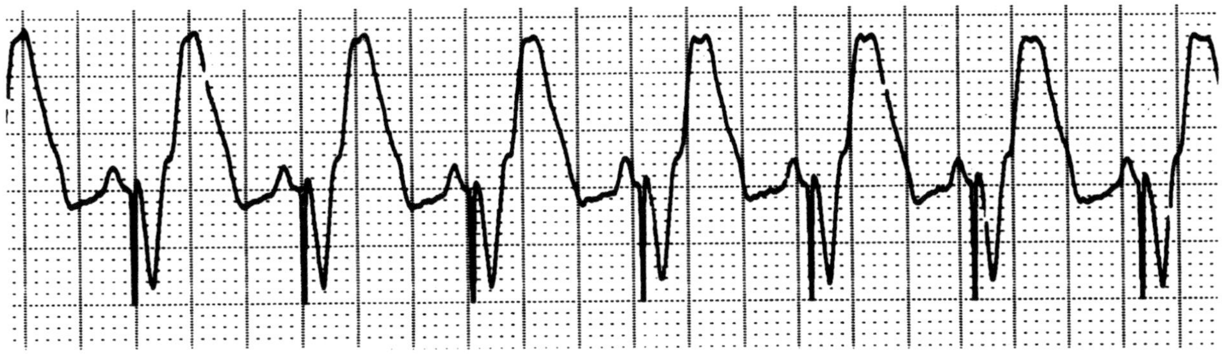

1. List all of the events noted on the tracing.
2. Is pacemaker function normal?
3. What is the atrial rate and what is the ventricular rate?

Sensed atrial
V- paced

Answer:

1. The following events occur on the tracing:
    Appropriate atrial sensing (**1**)
    Ventricular capture (**2**)

2. On first inspection the pacemaker function appears normal with P-synchronous pacing at or near the upper rate limit of 95 bpm. However, don't forget to keep all of the programmed parameters in mind. We are told that the sensed AV interval is 200 ms. In the tracing previously shown, the sensed AV interval appears to be approximately 120 ms, significantly shorter than 200 ms. Surface electrocardiograms can be misleading because there may be a significant difference between timing on the surface tracing and timing on the intracardiac tracing. However, a difference of 80 ms is unlikely. One must therefore suspect an abnormality.

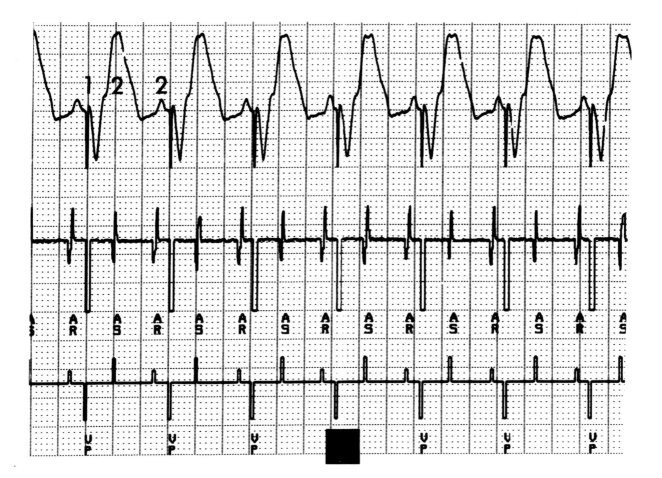

3. The atrial and ventricular rates appear to be approximately 95 bpm on the ECG tracing previously shown. However, the timing diagram demonstrates an atrial rate of approximately 190 bpm with every other atrial event occurring in the PVARP and therefore designated as a refractory event (**AR**). Every other atrial event (**S**) is a retrograde P wave and is the atrial event that triggers the AV interval followed by pseudo-Wenckebach prolongation of the AV interval until the upper rate limit times out at 95 bpm. The native atrial depolarization therefore occurs within the prolonged AV interval during which the atrial sensing circuit is refractory. The native atrial event is noted on the timing diagram as a refractory event (**R**).

COMPLEX

CASE 1

Question:

You are asked to see a patient with a ventricular-based DDDR pacemaker that is programmed to the following parameters:

Lower rate = 60 bpm
Maximum sensor rates = 140 bpm
PVARP = 200 ms
AVI = 175 ms

The referring physician was questioning whether the following ECGs were compatible with normal pacemaker function as programmed.

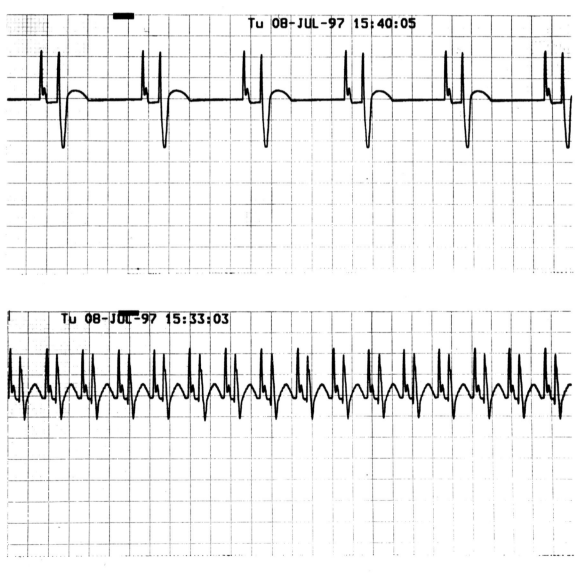

1. Is the pacemaker function normal?
2. Is reprogramming required?

Answer:

1. Pacemaker function is normal. As stated, this is a ventricular-based DDDR pacemaker. This means that timing occurs from the ventricular event. A pure ventricular-based timing system can result in a ventricular rate that is faster than the programmed rate limit.

The key to interpretation of the ECG is the fact that the patient has intrinsic AV conduction. The interval from the paced atrial event to the intrinsic QRS is approximately 105 ms. It is difficult to measure the exact AR interval on the surface ECG, but an exact measurement can be obtained from the ECG interpretation channel.

Consider the following equations:

$$VV = AV + VA$$
$$RR = AR + RA$$

Programmed VV = 140 bpm = 430 ms

430 - 175 = 255 ms = VA

In this case, the AV interval is abbreviated by faster conduction at 105 ms:

$$RR = AR + VA$$
$$RR = 105 \text{ ms} + 255 \text{ ms} = 360 \text{ ms} = 166 \text{ bpm}$$

The effective ventricular rate is 26 bpm faster than the programmed upper rate limit.

2. Whether or not programming changes are required depends on the patient and what rates can be clinically tolerated. In this particular patient, if it is believed that 140 bpm is the fastest rate the patient can tolerate, the VA interval can be lengthened by programming a longer PVARP. For example, a PVARP of 310 ms in this case would result in:

$$RR = 120 \text{ ms} + 310 \text{ ms} = 430 \text{ ms} = 140 \text{ bpm}$$

In most contemporary pacemakers, regardless of timing system, there is usually some modification of the pure ventricular-based timing operation, that corrects this potential aberrancy. For example, if the AV interval is abbreviated, the pacemaker may automatically add that interval to the VA interval to maintain the upper rate limit. Multiple variations of this exist. It is important to thoroughly understand the timing mechanisms of pacemakers that you implant and/or follow.

CASE 2

Question:

A young woman receives a DDDR pacemaker for hypertrophic obstructive cardiomyopathy that is refractory to aggressive medical therapy. To assess pacemaker function, an exercise test is obtained one month following pacemaker implantation. The pacemaker is programmed to the following parameters:

Lower rate:	60 bpm
Upper rate:	140 bpm
Sensed AV interval:	100 ms
Paced AV interval:	120 ms
PVARP:	230 ms

The following tracings were obtained during the exercise test and the point at which they were obtained is noted:

Resting ECG tracing

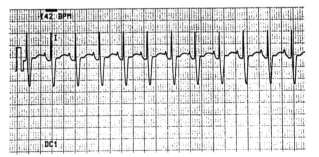

ECG tracing at 6 minutes/Bruce Protocol

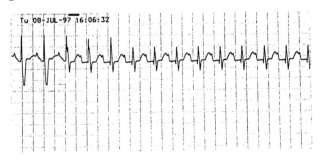

ECG tracing at 8 minutes/Bruce Protocol

1. Is pacemaker function normal during exercise?
2. Should any programming changes be made?

Answer:

1. Pacemaker function is normal. When the patient's intrinsic atrial rate exceeds the upper rate limit of 140 bpm (428 ms), pseudo-Wenckebach behavior occurs. However, in this patient with a normal conduction system, AV conduction occurs and results in an intrinsic QRS complex before the pseudo-Wenckebach AV interval has been terminated at the upper rate cycle length, 428 ms, by a paced ventricular beat.

2. The benefit derived by pacing in patients with hypertrophic obstructive cardiomyopathy is presumed to be due to altered ventricular activation sequence that results from right ventricular apical pacing. If there is no ventricular depolarization no benefit can be expected. Shortening the sensed AV interval will not help because the pacemaker would still respect the upper rate limit interval and pseudo-Wenckebach behavior would be seen. Options would include raising the maximum tracking limit and/or programming "on" a rate-adaptive AV interval. At the current TARP, the maximum tracking limit is limited to approximately 140 bpm. If the sensed AV interval shortened to 60 ms at maximum exercise, the TARP would be 290 ms or potential maximum tracking limit of > 200 bpm.

CASE 3

Question:

Pacemaker parameters:

DDD
Lower Raté   50 bpm
Upper Rate   100 bpm
AV interval   150 ms
PVARP   300 ms

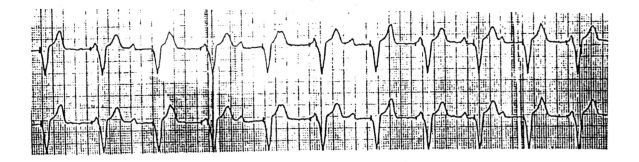

Why are some P waves followed by the paced QRS complexes and others are not? Is this normal DDD function?

Answer:

There are P waves (**solid squares**) which are not tracked even though they are not at upper rate. On the other hand, these P waves are followed by a paced ventricular event. Therefore, in DDD, one explanation would be undersensing of the P waves indicated by the solid squares with oversensing resulting in tracking. However, it would be too fortuitous that these oversensed atrial events occurred at similar times. One explanation would be that the mode is actually DDI or DDIR. How would this occur? Some devices "mode-switch" in response to rapid atrial events to the DDI or DDIR mode. Atrial oversensing, such as caused by electromagnetic interference, might cause mode switching to DDIR. The black arrows indicate the paced ventricular events and the four-point stars indicate the atrial paced events.

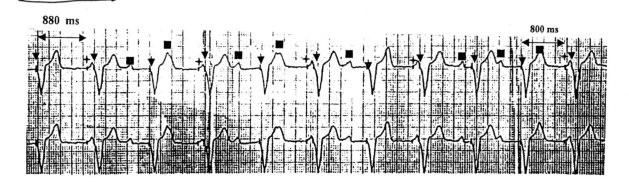

CASE 4

Question:

A patient is referred to you because the patient's primary physician does not believe that the rhythm strip obtained is his office could be compatible with normal function. You are told that the patient's DDI pacemaker is programmed to a lower rate of 86 bpm, AV delay of 225 ms, and a ventricular blanking period of 10 ms. The following rhythm strip is sent with the patient: *165*

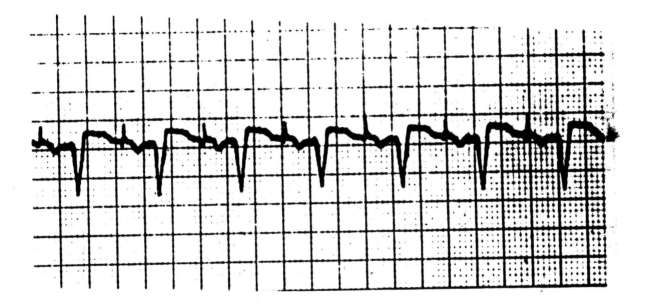

1. Is this compatible with normal DDI function?
2. What programming changes would be appropriate?

Answer:

1. The tracing is not compatible with normal DDI function. The tracing reveals an AR interval longer than the programmed AV interval and a rate of approximately 96 bpm which is faster than the programmed rate of the pacemaker. The following calculations can be used to solve this electrocardiographic abnormality:

VV = AV + VA
VV - AV = VA
VV = 86 bpm = 697 ms
AV = 165 ms
Measured RR = 575 ms
697 ms - 165 ms = 532 ms = UA\
575 ms - 532 ms = 43 ms
   RR   UA

Point of sensing after atrial output is 43 ms at which point the VA interval is initiated; when VA interval of 532 ms is completed, another atrial output is delivered.

2. Lengthening the blanking period to 43 ms should avoid crosstalk. After this programming change the following tracing was obtained. This tracing now conforms to the programmed parameters with an AV interval of 165 ms and a rate of 86 bpm.

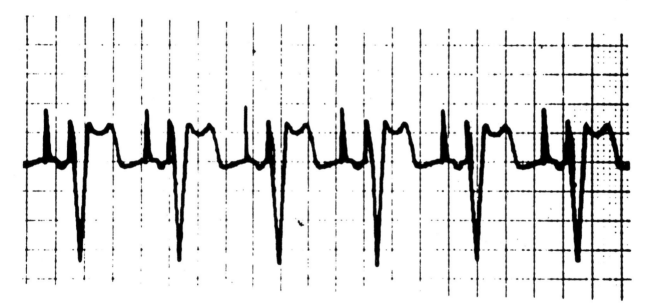

CASE 5

Question:

A 10-year-old girl with a DDD pacemaker implanted elsewhere is referred for evaluation with subjective complaints of an "arrhythmia." She has had a modified-Fontan procedure and originally received a VVI pacemaker but had severe pacemaker syndrome. The atrial lead is transvenous and there are multiple epicardial ventricular leads. The pacemaker is programmed to the following parameters:

Mode:	DDDR
Lower rate:	85 bpm 705 ms
Upper rate:	152 BPM 394 ms
AV delay:	180 ms
Ventricular pulse width:	1.2 ms
Ventricular voltage amplitude:	6.0 V
Atrial pulse width:	1.6 ms
Atrial voltage amplitude:	6.0 V
PVARP:	275 ms
Blanking period:	38 ms
Ventricular safety pacing option:	On
Ventricular refractory period:	250 ms

VA = 525 ms

Atrial and ventricular thresholds were as follows:

Ventricular:	7.0 V at 0.2 ms pulse width
Atrial:	3.0 V at 0.2 ms pulse width

A rhythm strip during the patient's subjective complaints of "arrhythmia" follows:

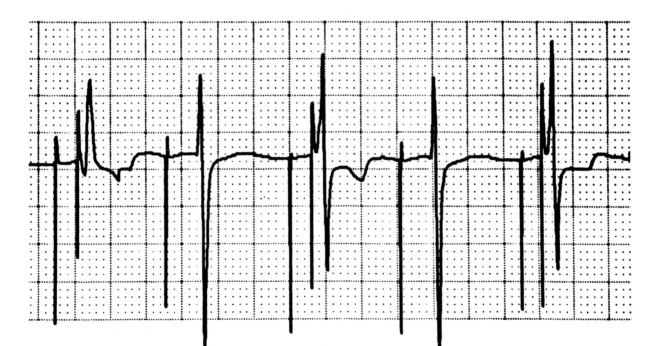

1. Is there any apparent explanation for the frequent safety pacing?
2. Should any programming changes be made?

Answer:

1. The atrial outputs are programmed much higher than necessary given the thresholds. Safety pacing occurs when there is sensing in the crosstalk-sensing window, the interval immediately following the ventricular blanking period (**arrows**). At other times there is intrinsic conduction through the AV node followed by an intrinsic QRS complex (**asterisks**). The measured AR interval is approximately 220 ms which is longer than the programmed AV interval. Although electrograms or an ECG diagnostic channel would be required for absolute proof, it is possible that the atrial output in these cycles is sensed after the cross-talk sensing window, and inhibits ventricular output. Because the patient has intact AV conduction, one sees a prolonged AR followed by QRS as opposed to ventricular asystole which would occur if the patient was pacemaker dependent.

When the atrial output was decreased, safety pacing was no longer seen.

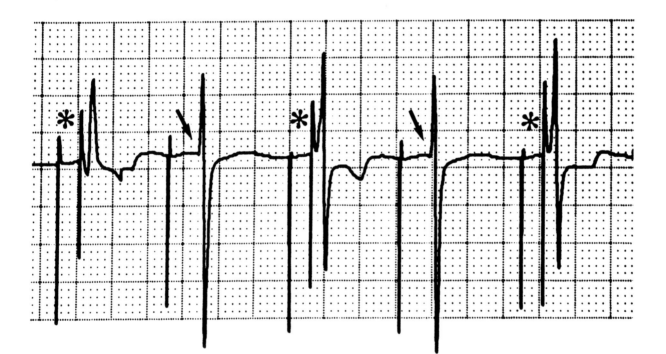

2. The appropriate programming change in this patient would be to permanently lower the atrial output. If atrial thresholds required such high outputs then some other programming solution would have to be sought. One would be to extend the ventricular blanking period. The potential negative effect of prolonging the blanking period would be the potential for true ventricular activity to occur in the blanking period and not be sensed which could result in competitive ventricular pacing.

The ventricular thresholds are very high consistent with the patient's new epicardial ventricular pacing leads. Transvenous ventricular leads were not a possibility due to the patient's congenital cardiac anomalies.

CASE 6

Question:

Programmed Settings:

DDD
Lower Rate   45 bpm (1333ms)
Upper Rate   160 bpm (375ms)
AV Delay   130 ms
PVARP   270 ms
Rate Drop   ON
Bottom Rate   45 bpm
Intervention rate 100 bpm

VA =1203

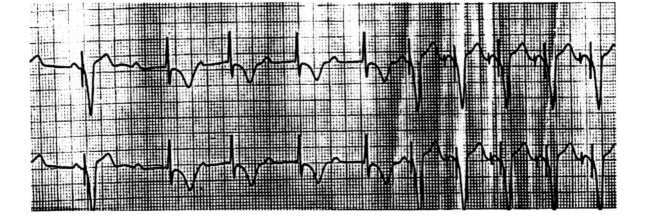

What is the likely cause(s) of the abnormality?

Answer:

Programmed Settings:

DDD
Lower Rate	45 bpm (1333ms)
Upper Rate	160 bpm (375ms)
AV Delay	130 ms
PVARP	270 ms
Rate Drop	ON
Bottom Rate	45 bpm
Intervention Rate	100 bpm

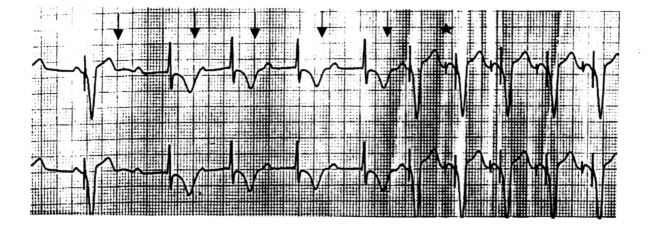

The first beat on the left is a P wave followed by a ventricular paced event at the appropriate AV delay. However, the next P wave is not followed by a ventricular paced event. Since the P is beyond the PVARP, the two most likely explanations are atrial undersensing or ventricular oversensing. If the phenomenon was the result of electromagnetic interference, ventricular oversensing (timing of ventricular sensed events is indicated by arrows) would be the likely diagnosis. Ventricular oversensing may result in apparent atrial undersensing since the P waves fall within the PVARP of the ventricular oversensed events. In either case, the atrial rate is felt to be slower than the lower rate but since there are ventricular sensed events above this rate, there is no AV pacing following these P waves.

The rapid rate of AV pacing is at the rate drop rate of 100bpm (onset of rate drop indicated by a star). Why does rate drop occur? Rate drop occurs when programmed "ON" and the atrial rate decreases below the programmed bottom rate of 45 bpm. What is the mode during rate drop? The mode remains the programmed mode, in this case DDD. Other causes of AV pacing at a rate faster than the lower rate include rate smoothing and rate adaptive pacing.

CASE 7

Question:

A pacemaker was implanted for intermittent AV block. Two weeks later the patient had apparent atrial undersensing and was told the atrial lead should be replaced. A second procedure was done. Several weeks later he was again told that there was a problem with the atrial lead and it should be replaced again. The patient comes for a second opinion. During the initial pacemaker clinic evaluation there is evidence of gross atrial undersensing. This is corrected by programming to a more sensitive atrial channel. An ambulatory monitor was then obtained to be certain that the atrial undersensing had been corrected. The gross atrial undersensing that was previously seen was no longer present but the following tracing was noted on the Holter. (Arrows note "P" waves.)

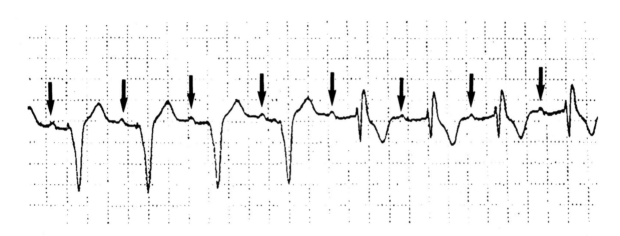

At the time of the Holter, programmed settings were as follows:

Mode:	DDD
Lower Rate:	60 bpm
Upper Rate:	120 bpm
Sensed AV delay:	120 ms
Paced AV delay:	170 ms
PVARP:	250 ms
PVARP Extension:	On
Pulse width:	0.5 ms in both chambers
Atrial voltage amplitude:	3.5 V
Ventricular voltage amplitude:	4.0 V
Blanking period:	38 ms
Ventricular refractory period:	220 ms

A-rate 88

1. Are these tracings compatible with normal function?
2. Would you make any programming changes?

Answer:

1. In the tracing on the preceding page, initially there is normal P wave sensing followed by a paced ventricular beat. The latter portion of the tracing reveals continued sinus activity but there is a longer PR interval, greater than the programmed AV interval, and an intrinsic QRS complex follows.

This represents functional atrial undersensing. The pacemaker is intermittently sensing a T wave. (See tracings below.) Sensing a ventricular event followed by sensing of the T wave on the ventricular channel is recognized by the pacemaker as 2 consecutive ventricular events without an intervening atrial event. This satisfies the pacemaker's definition of a PVC and per programmed settings, the PVARP is extended following a PVC. When extended, the PVARP is 480 ms. Extension of the PVARP results in the next P wave falling in the PVARP and since no atrial event is sensed, the PVARP is continually extended until a P wave falls outside of the extended PVARP.

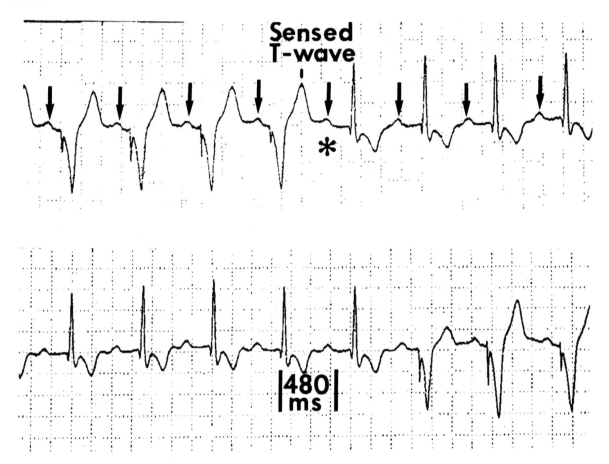

2. Several programming options exist. The PVARP extension can be programmed off. Alternatively, the ventricular sensing circuit could be made less sensitive to avoid sensing the T wave.

CASE 8

Question:

A 66-year-old male presents with pacemaker syndrome following DDDR pacemaker placement. Pacemaker syndrome occurred because of ventricular tracking of myopotentials. During these episodes the patient effectively had VVIR pacing, and the loss of AV synchrony resulted in symptoms. Programmed parameters were as follows:

Lower rate:	50 bpm
Upper rate:	120 bpm
Voltage:	3.5 volts in both chambers
PW:	0.45 ms in both chambers
Paced AV Interval:	200 ms
PVARP:	250 ms
Sensed AV Interval:	150 ms
Pacing configuration:	Unipolar
Sensing configuration:	Unipolar
Sensitivity:	A = 0.8 mV and V = 3.5 mV
PVARP = 200	
CVTL = 85	

↑pRP 450 ns

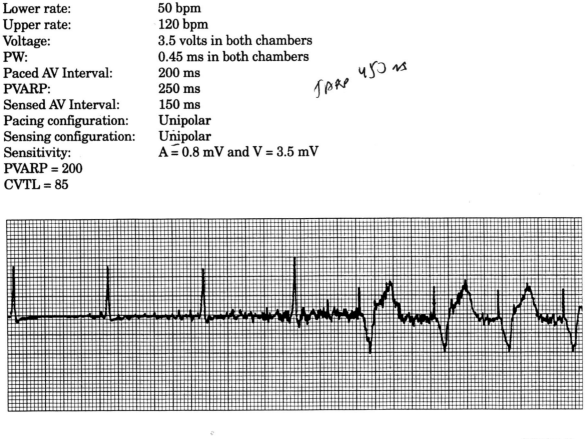

CM721311L.58

Rhythm strip during symptoms:

1. What determines at what rate the myopotential activity will be tracked?
2. In this case, the upper rate is programmed to 120 bpm, 500 ms, which is not the same as the TARP. Does this discrepancy in any way effect the upper rate limit and the myopotential tracking in this case?

↓VARP

Answer:

1. Tracking any electromagnetic interference or tracking an atrial tachyarrhythmia depends on several factors. The most important factors include the amplitude of the signal being sensed. If large enough, the extracardiac signal would be sensed consistently. In most pacemakers, the pacemaker's rate response depends largely on the programmed upper rate limit. In the programmed parameters there is a feature designated "CVTL" that is programmed "on." This abbreviation denotes Conditional Ventricular Tracking Limit. This feature can effect the upper rate limit. The pacemaker will limit tracking to 35 beats faster than the lower rate limit unless the activity sensor indicates a faster rate. This "cross-checking" between the sensor and intrinsic cardiac activity is responsible for the paced ventricular rate response to the atrial myopotentials. The patient's response to the myopotential signals is explained by CVTL. The patient's lower rate, 50 bpm plus 35 bpm, or 85 bpm, determines the rate limit as long as the activity sensor does not indicated higher rates.

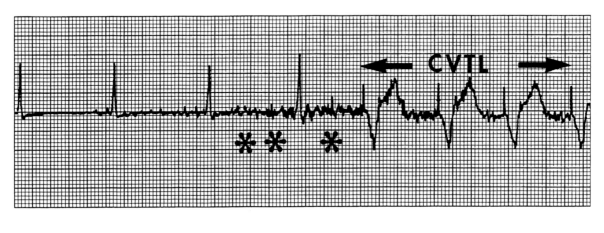

CM721311L.58

2. In this case the paced response during the myopotential activity (**asterisks**) is explained by the CVTL. This is not effected by the programmed upper rate limit or the TARP. The fact that there is a discrepancy between the URL and the TARP is not significant. When the upper rate is reached, the slower of these 2 values defines the upper rate limit. For example, this patient would be limited to 120 bpm, the programmed upper rate limit. Most current dual-chamber pacemakers would not allow an upper rate limit that is faster than that defined by the TARP to be programmed. However, if allowed by the pacemaker, e.g. URL 150 and TARP of 450 ms or 133 bpm, the TARP would effectively define the URL.

CASE 9

Question:

A 76-year-old male with sinus node dysfunction and pacemaker implantation four years earlier is found to have intermittent ventricular undersensing during routine trans-telephonic transmission. The patient returns for further evaluation. The chest x-ray is shown:

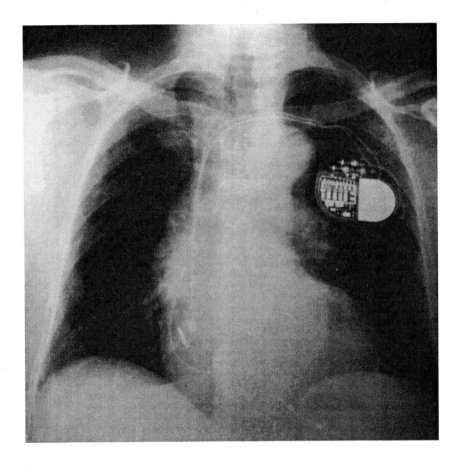

1. Describe the pacing system by trying to detect as many details as possible from the chest x-ray.
2. Can your clinical suspicions be confirmed by the chest x-ray?
3. What would you advise?

Answer:

1. The chest x-ray demonstrates a dual-chamber pacemaker. Close inspection of the leads and the connector block reveals the atrial lead and connector block to be bipolar. The ventricular lead and connection is actually "tripolar." The "3rd" pole of the ventricular lead was utilized for a special rate-adaptive sensor which was located within the lead. The pacemaker is in a prepectoral position. Lead position appears adequate in terms of intracardiac positioning. The leads have been placed via the subclavian vein and there is distinct "kinking" of the leads as they pass between the clavicle and the first rib. This radiographic appearance is worrisome for the potential development of "crush injury" to the leads. In this patient there was crush injury with insulation damage which presented as a sensing abnormality.

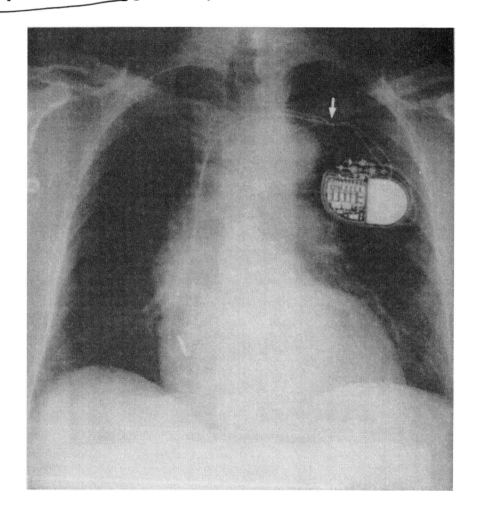

2. The clinical history is compatible with ventricular lead failure due to insulation defect. Sensing abnormalities are the most common manifestation of lead insulation failure. Determining the lead impedance may lend additional confirmatory evidence of the presence of an insulation defect. Insulation failure would result in a very low measured impedance. However, failure to record a low impedance does not rule out the presence of an insulation defect. Sometimes multiple impedance determinations and/or repetitive impedance measurements while manipulating the pacemaker pocket/connector block and/or the patients ipsilateral upper extremity may also bring out the low impedance value by stressing the lead.

The actual insulation defects cannot usually be detected by chest x-ray. However, subclavian "kinking" of the lead should raise suspicion for possible lead abnormalities. Insulation indentations from ligatures placed around the anchoring sleeve can often be seen, but these do not translate to insulation damage.

CASE 10

Question:

Pacemaker Programmed Settings:

Mode	DDD
Lower Rate	60 bpm (1000 ms)
Upper Rate	120 bpm (500 ms)
AV Delay	140 ms (paced, sensed)
PVARP	310 ms

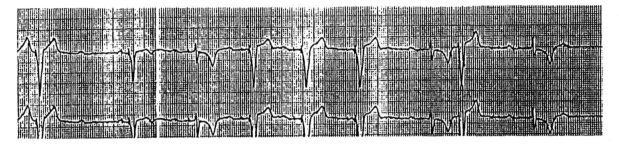

Electromagnetic interference resulted in these findings. What types of abnormalities are seen?

paced v E. caple
~~Sento~~
native p wove S v- tracks

native p, long AV, native QRS

v- oversensing

Answer:

The first beat on the left is a paced ventricular complex. Next there is a P wave (**star**) which is undersensed. Undersensing of the P wave may be due to a low amplitude atrial signal , an R wave which is oversensed placing the P wave in the PVARP, or a noise reversion mode. The atrial escape interval (the lower rate interval minus the A-V delay = 1000 ms – 140 ms) of 860 ms indicates that a paced atrial event should have occurred at the end of this interval. The most likely explanation is that an oversensed ventricular event (**solid arrow pointing up**) occurred, so that 860 ms later at the end of the atrial escape interval a paced atrial event occurs. The second P wave (**star**) is not sensed. This may be due to the onset of a noise reversion mode, usually DOO, when the programmed mode is DDD, or so-called 'late sensing" of the P wave, because the onset of the local atrial electrogram has not yet occurred. The third, fourth, and fifth P waves (**stars**) are not tracked as expected in the DDD mode (the P waves are outside the PVARP). This "undersensing" of these P waves is due to the noise reversion mode of DOO. At the end of noise reversion, another oversensed ventricular event (**solid arrow pointing up**) may occur, placing the sixth P wave (**star**) within the PVARP of 310 ms. At the right side of the panel, noise reversion again occurs, resulting in undersensing of the seventh P wave. However, the atrial paced event (**white arrow**) is not followed by a paced ventricular event. This is due to an unusual form of noise reversion, in which ventricular sensing within the AV interval inhibits output of the paced ventricular event. This occurs a second time at the next white arrow.

Thus, this is a case of oversensing in the ventricle resulting in P waves occurring in the PVARP and noise reversion.

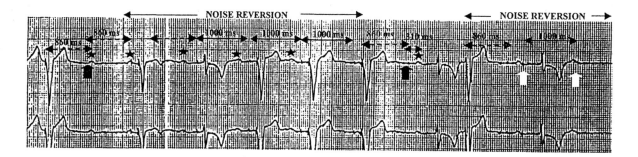